كاظم

FRCS: MCQs in
Applied Basic Sciences

FRCS: MCQs in Applied Basic Sciences

L.D. Wijesinghe MA, MB, BChir,
P.A. Sylvester MB, ChB
and K.S. Cheng MA, MB, BChir
Demonstrators in Anatomy, University of Cambridge, UK

With a Foreword by Professor Harold Ellis CBE, FRCS

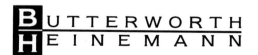

Butterworth-Heinemann Ltd
Linacre House, Jordan Hill, Oxford OX2 8DP

$\mathcal{R}$ A member of the Reed Elsevier plc group

OXFORD   LONDON   BOSTON
MUNICH   NEW DELHI   SINGAPORE   SYDNEY
TOKYO   TORONTO   WELLINGTON

First published 1993
Reprinted 1994

© Butterworth-Heinemann Ltd 1993

British Library Cataloguing in Publication Data
Wijesinghe, Lasantha
    FRCS: MCQs in Applied Basic Science
    I. Title   II. Sylvester, Paul
    III. Cheng, Koon Soong
    610.76
ISBN 0 7506 0986 9

Typeset by TecSet Ltd, Wallington, Surrey
Printed and bound in Great Britain by
Biddles Ltd, Guildford and King's Lynn

Contents

Foreword

I was an Examiner in Anatomy in the Primary FRCS when multiple choice questions (MCQs) were first introduced. Nowadays, whether you like them or not, they are here to stay as an established part of the examination system. They have the obvious advantage that every candidate is asked exactly the same set of questions and also that they can be marked dispassionately by the computer!

Every type of examination requires careful preparation by the candidate. It is with the candidate for Part I of the FRCS in mind that the authors have put together this small but extremely useful volume. Not only does it contain helpful advice about how to approach MCQs in the Basic Science Examination of the Royal College of Surgeons, and a large selection of typical MCQ questions (and their correct answers), but also there are valuable hints on the oral part of the examination with a selection of genuine *viva voce* questions.

I have no doubt that surgeons in training will benefit from a careful study of this book. I believe it has the great advantage that its authors have themselves all been through the mill of this examination and write with the warm passion of recent (and successful!) candidates.

Professor Harold Ellis CBE, FRCS
Clinical Anatomist
University of Cambridge

Preface

The Primary Examination of the Royal College of Surgeons has undergone a change in its style and emphasis in recent times. Previous books of MCQs have not given the candidate much guidance in preparing for the examination or in approaching its separate sections.

For the above reasons we have included explanatory notes on the format of the examination and practical hints on sitting the different sections.

The viva has always been a stumbling block to many. This book contains sample viva questions taken verbatim from candidates – a feature which is not present in other books of this type.

The book is in three main sections. The first sets out MCQs in anatomy, physiology and pharmacology, and pathology. The second is a sample MCQ paper, and the third is a section of viva questions.

We wish to thank Professor Harold Ellis, Dr Chris Huang and Dr Derek Wight who have looked over the questions in detail. In addition, Mr Bari Logan and his staff in the Department of Anatony at Cambridge have given us a great deal of support and encouragement during the writing of this book.

LDW
PAS
KSC
Cambridge,
November 1992

The format of the examination

The Applied Basic Sciences examination of the Royal College of Surgeons of England is in two sections. The first section consists of 90 MCQs of the format shown in this book. There are 30 questions in each of the disciplines of anatomy, pathology and physiology. Included in the physiology section are some questions in clinical pharmacology. The emphasis of the questions is that of basic sciences as applied to clinical surgery.

If you reach the required standard in the MCQ section you will be invited to attend the viva section of the examination. There are six vivas, two in each of the disciplines. Each viva lasts 10 minutes and is conducted by two examiners. One of these is a clinician and the other is a 'basic scientist'. One examiner will ask the questions while the other scores your performance. The first anatomy viva is preceded by a 10 minute period for the interpretation of histology slides.

The examinations of the Colleges of Glasgow and Edinburgh are broadly similar but the viva is a 20 minute session in anatomy. There are no vivas in physiology or pathology.

You will be scored in the MCQ and each viva as follows: a mark of 12 or more is a pass whereas 10 or 11 are below the required standard. To pass you need to score usually at least 36 in each discpline, e.g. 12 in the MCQ, 12 in the first viva and 12 in the second or 11, 12, 13, or any combination which adds up to 36.

If you are successful your candidate number will be announced at the end of the day and you will be invited to join the examiners for a glass of wine. You can then complain that the examination was far too easy

How to prepare for the examination

For most candidates this will be their first postgraduate professional examination. Many fail because they are poorly prepared and do not know what is expected of them. Familiarize yourself with the format of the examination which is described in this book and you will be one step ahead of the rest.

Your next task is to gain a solid grounding in basic surgical science. The recommended texts and references are useful, but so is your clinical experience. There are many courses run at centres throughout the country which prepare candidates for the examination. Several of our colleagues have found these useful, especially in getting to grips with prosected anatomical specimens. We gained from our time as Anatomy Demonstrators at the University of Cambridge. Teaching anatomy to medical students under the auspices of a mentor such as Harold Ellis is the surest way of learning the subject thoroughly. Other centres such as Bristol include some teaching in physiology and pathology.

Armed with your knowledge and experience you will be able to approach the MCQs. This method of examination will be unfamiliar to some candidates but can be mastered with adequate practice. Do as many MCQs as possible and aim to get over 60% correct. You will find this difficult to begin with but persevere; your effort will be rewarded.

Having passed the MCQ paper your next hurdle is the viva section. Here the knowledge you have gained from books, courses and clinical experience must be retrieved and presented to the examiner in a cogent and confident manner. Practise this with colleagues. Ask each other sample viva questions and then criticize the answers so that all may learn. Alternatively, choose a subject at random from the index of a textbook and try to talk coherently about that topic for a minute or longer. Pick up a bone such as the humerus or fibula and impress your friends with a dissertation on its anatomical features. In this way you will become used to answering questions out loud.

Familiarize yourself with the microscopy of normal histological sections, in particular, gut, skin, vas deferens, ureter and muscle of all types. You are asked to identify three slides as part of the anatomy viva.

Be confident in identifying anatomical structures on prosected specimens. Revise surface anatomy on a consenting friend and make sure you can perform a slick examination of the cranial nerves and large joints. You may be called upon to demonstrate surface anatomy in the vivas, either on yourself (e.g. anatomical snuff box) or on a live model.

These simple guidelines will help you through various stages of the examination. Above all, never argue with the examiners and never attempt to be familiar with them. This is a serious professional examination.

If you are well-prepared you are likely to pass, but there is no guarantee of success. Many of the consultant surgeons you work for will have failed some part of the Fellowship Examination.

Finally, ensure that you spend as much effort on physiology and pathology as you do on anatomy. Past experience shows that when candidates fail, they fail most often in physiology!

Recommended texts and references

Anatomy

Agur A.M.R. (1990) *Grant's Atlas of Anatomy*, 9th edn. Williams & Wilkins, Baltimore.

Basmajian J.V. (1989) *Grant's Method of Anatomy*, 11th edn. Williams & Wilkins, Baltimore.

Ellis H. (1992) *Clinical Anatomy*, 8th edn. Blackwell Scientific, Oxford.

McMinn R.M.H. (1990) *Last's Anatomy Regional and Applied*, 8th edn. Churchill Livingstone, Edinburgh.

Williams P.L. *et al.* (eds) (1989) *Gray's Anatomy*, 37th edn. Churchill Livingstone, Edinburgh.

Physiology

Ganong W. F. (1991) *Review of Medical Physiology*, 15th edn. Appleton & Lange, Englewood Cliffs, New Jersey.

Guyton A.C. (1991) *Textbook of Human Physiology*, 8th edn. WB Saunders, Philadelphia.

Lamb J.F. *et al.* (1991) *Essentials of Physiology*, 3rd edn. Blackwell Scientific, Oxford.

Pathology

Gardner & Tweedle (1989) *Pathology for Primary FRCS*. Edward Arnold, London.

Thomas C.G.A. (1983) *Medical Microbiology*, 6th edn. Bailliere Tindall, Baltimore.

Walter J.B. and Israel M.S. (1989) *General Pathology*, 6th edn. Churchill Livingstone, Edinburgh.

Wolf N. (1986) *Cell, Tissue and Disease: The Basis of Pathology*, 2nd edn. WB Saunders, Philadelphia.

Anatomy MCQs

Head and neck

1. The tongue—
   a. The tip drains unilaterally to the submental nodes
   b. The anterior two-thirds develops in part from the tuberculum impar
   c. The hypoglossus muscle protrudes the tongue
   d. The vallate papillae lie anterior to the sulcus terminalis
   e. The hypoglossal nerve supplies all the muscles both intrinsic and extrinsic

2. The tongue—
   a. Is divided into an anterior third and a posterior two-thirds by the sulcus terminalis
   b. Contains intrinsic muscles derived from the occipital mytomes
   c. Contains the foramen caecum, which marks the beginning of the thyroglossal duct
   d. Receives parasympathetic secretomotor fibres from the otic ganglion in its posterior third part
   e. Contains circumvallate taste buds, which are innervated by the chorda tympani

3. The parotid gland—
   a. Lies within an easily distensible capsule
   b. Is in contact with the osseous part of the external auditory canal
   c. Secretomotor supply is from the pterygopalatine ganglion
   d. Is traversed by the internal carotid artery
   e. Contains lymph nodes

4. In the orbital cavity—
   a. The superior orbital fissure transmits the fourth and sixth cranial nerves
   b. The optic canal transmits the ophthalmic artery
   c. The ciliary ganglion lies on the medial side of the optic nerve
   d. The nerve to the inferior oblique contains parasympathetic as well as motor fibres
   e. The frontal nerve lies between levator palpebrae superioris and superior rectus muscles

Answers overleaf

1. b. d.

The tongue is developed from the first, third and fourth pharyngeal arches. The anterior two-thirds is formed from the two lingual swellings of the first arch and the tuberculum impar. The posterior third is formed from the hypobranchial eminence of the third arch with a small contribution from the fourth arch. The tip drains bilaterally to the submental nodes. The hypoglossus muscle depresses and retracts the tongue with the genioglossus muscle protruding the tongue. The hypoglossal nerve does not supply the palatoglossus muscle; this is supplied by the vagus nerve.

2. b. c. d.

The tongue is divided into anterior two-thirds and a posterior third by the sulcus terminalis.

Although the circumvallate papillae lie in front of the sulcus terminalis, they are innervated by the glossopharyngeal nerve.

3. b. e.

The capsule of the parotid gland is formed from the investing layer of cervical fascia. It is not distensible and so generalized swelling of the parotid, e.g. mumps, causes pain. The gland is in contact with both the osseous and cartilaginous parts of the external auditory canal. The secretomotor supply is by the auriculotemporal nerve which contains fibres from the otic ganglion. The external carotid artery and retromandibular vein traverse the gland. Members of the preauricular group of lymph nodes lie within and on the gland.

4. a. b. d.

The ciliary ganglion lies below and lateral to the optic nerve.

The frontal nerve lies between the orbital plate of the frontal bone above and the levator palpebrae superior muscle below.

5. **In the orbit—**
   a. The medial rectus is supplied by the abducens nerve
   b. The trochlear nerve supplies the inferior oblique muscle
   c. The sphincter pupillae is supplied from the Edinger–Westphal nucleus
   d. The lesser wing of the sphenoid forms part of the roof
   e. The ophthalmic artery is a direct branch of the internal carotid artery

6. **In the neck—**
   a. The sternomastoid muscle is the principal rotator of the atlanto-occipital joint
   b. Damage to the accessory nerve (XI) results in winged scapula
   c. C3 is level with the upper border of the thyroid cartilage
   d. The facial artery runs deep to the posterior belly of the digastric muscle
   e. The great auricular nerve ascends deep to sternomastoid

7. **At the root of the neck—**
   a. The scalenus medius attaches to the scalene tubercle
   b. The phrenic nerve descends posterior to the subclavian vein
   c. The thoracic duct passes posterior to the carotid sheath
   d. The inferior thyroid artery crosses posterior to the sympathetic trunk
   e. The cords of the brachial plexus emerge posterior to scalenus anterior

8. **At the level of the 6th cervical vertebra (C6)—**
   a. The common carotid artery bifurcates into the external and internal carotid arteries
   b. The superior thyroid vein drains into the internal jugular vein
   c. The middle thyroid vein drains into the internal jugular vein
   d. The roots of the phrenic nerve unite together at the lateral border of scalenus anterior
   e. Lies the isthmus of the thyroid gland

Answers overleaf

5. c. d. e.
The medial rectus is supplied by the oculomotor nerve and the trochlear nerve supplies the superior oblique. The roof of the orbit is formed anteriorly by the orbital plates of the frontal bone, and posteriorly by the lesser wing of the sphenoid.

6. a. d.
Damage to the accessory nerve causes dropped shoulder by paralysing trapezius. The upper border of the thyroid cartilage is at the level of C4. The great auricular nerve ascends superficial to sternomastoid and is therefore at risk in operations on the neck.

7. b. d.
Scalenus anterior attaches to the scalene tubercle. The phrenic nerve usually crosses posterior to the subclavian vein but may pass anteriorly or even through the vein! The cords of the brachial plexus lie in the posterior triangle of the neck, but the trunks emerge posterior to scalenus anterior.

8. c. d.
The common carotid artery bifurcates at the level of the upper border of the thyroid cartilage corresponding to C4.

The isthmus of the thyroid gland usually lies in front of the second, third and fourth tracheal rings.

9. **The temporomandibular joint—**
   a. Contains a disc of hyaline cartilage
   b. Is supplied by the great auricular nerve
   c. Is usually dislocated posteriorly
   d. Protraction is by the medial pterygoid muscle
   e. Is most stable when the mouth is half-open

10. **The thyroid gland—**
    a. Has an isthmus which lies anterior to the second, third and fourth tracheal rings
    b. Has an isthmus which receives its blood supply from the thyroidea ima artery
    c. May be found in the posterior third of the tongue
    d. Is supplied usually by both the subclavian and the external carotid arteries
    e. May be connected to the hyoid bone by levator glandulae thyroidae

11. **The larynx—**
    a. Has the lateral cricoarytenoid as an adductor of the vocal cord
    b. Has the posterior cricoarytenoid as an adductor of the vocal cord
    c. Has the vocal ligament as the upper part of the cricothyroid membrane
    d. Has an inlet, which is guarded by the oblique arytenoid muscles
    e. Has a rima glottidis, which is the opening between the two vocal folds

12. **The middle meatus of the nasal cavity—**
    a. Contains the bulla ethmoidalis formed by the anterior ethmoidal sinus
    b. Contains the hiatus semilunaris above the bulla
    c. Contain the hiatus semilunaris, the anterior end of which receives the infundibulum
    d. Receives the drainage of the maxillary sinus
    e. Receives the drainage of the posterior ethmoidal sinus

Answers overleaf

9. All false

The temporomandibular joint contains a disc of fibrocartilage and is supplied by the auriculotemporal nerve and the nerve to masseter. Dislocation usually occurs anteriorly. Protraction is brought about by the lateral pterygoids. The joint is most stable when the mouth is shut.

10. All

The thyroidea ima artery may arise from either the brachiocephalic trunk or the aortic arch.

Levator glandulae thyroidae is a muscular connection between the pyramidal lobe of the isthmus of the gland and the hyoid bone.

If the thyroid gland does not descend during its development, then it can be found in the posterior third of the tongue as lingual thyroid.

The thyroid gland is usually supplied by the superior thyroid artery (a branch of the external carotid artery) and the inferior thyroid artery (a branch of the thyrocervical trunk of the first part of the subclavian artery).

11. a. c. d. e.

The posterior cricoarytenoid is an abductor of the vocal cord.

12. c. d.

The bulla ethmoidalis is formed by the middle ethmoidal sinus. The hiatus semilunaris lies below the bulla. The posterior ethmoidal sinus drains into the superior meatus.

13. **The first pharyngeal (branchial) arch—**
    a. Gives rise to the malleus and the incus
    b. Is innervated by the trigeminal nerve
    c. Gives rise to the palatine tonsil
    d. Gives rise to the muscles of facial expression
    e. Gives rise to the external auditory meatus

14. **The oculomotor (third cranial) nerve—**
    a. Supplies the four recti muscles
    b. Divides into the superior and the inferior branches, which pass through the superior orbital fissure
    c. Carries parasympathetic fibres
    d. Supplies the levator palpebrae superioris muscle
    e. Supplies the orbicularis oculi muscle

15. **The trigeminal (fifth cranial) nerve—**
    a. Gives off the ophthalmic, maxillary and mandibular branches, which lie in the lateral wall of the cavernous sinus
    b. Supplies sensation to the tip of the nose
    c. Gives off the mandibular branch, which passes through the foramen ovale
    d. Gives off the maxillary branch, which passes through the foramen ovale
    e. Supplies sensory nerves to the entire face

16. **The facial (seventh cranial) nerve—**
    a. Carries parasympathetic secretomotor fibres to the parotid gland
    b. Has its motor nucleus in the pons
    c. Forms the pes anserinus
    d. Carries taste fibres from the anterior two-thirds of the tongue
    e. Gives off a branch to the tensor tympani muscle before it emerges out of the skull through the stylomastoid foramen

Answers overleaf

13. a. b. e.
The palatine tonsil is derived from the second pharyngeal (branchial) pouch. The muscles of facial expression are derived from the second pharyngeal (branchial) arch. They are innervated by the nerve of the second arch, i.e. the facial (seventh cranial) nerve.

14. b. c. d.
With the exception of the lateral rectus muscle (which is supplied by the abducens nerve), all the other recti are supplied by the oculomotor nerve.

The orbicularis oculi muscle is supplied by the facial nerve.

15. b. c.
Only the ophthalmic and maxillary branches are located in the lateral wall of the cavernous sinus.

The tip of the nose is supplied by the external nasal nerve, the terminal part of the anterior ethmoidal branch of the nasociliary nerve.

The maxillary nerve passes through the foramen rotundum.

The trigeminal nerve supplies sensation to the face except for an area over the angle of the mandible, which is supplied by the great auricular nerve (C2–3, cervical plexus).

16. b. c. d.
The facial nerve carries parasympathetic secretomotor fibres to the submandibular and sublingual glands. It is the glossopharyngeal (ninth cranial) nerve which carries parasympathetic secretomotor fibres to the parotid gland. The facial nerve gives off a branch to the stapedius muscle and also the chorda tympani branch, before it emerges through the stylomastoid foramen.

17.   The vagus nerve—
   a.   Emerges from the medulla oblongata between the pyramid and the olive
   b.   Gives off the recurrent laryngeal nerve on the right side as it passes over the first part of the subclavian artery
   c.   Contains nerve fibres from the nucleus ambiguus
   d.   Contains C1 nerve fibres
   e.   Supplies all the laryngeal muscles

Answers overleaf

17. b. c. e.

Vagus nerve emerges between the olive and the inferior cerebellar peduncle. Only the hypoglossal nerve emerges between the pyramid and the olive. Also the hypoglossal nerve contains fibres from C1 segment, which leave the nerve as the descendens hypoglossi to join the descending branch (C2 and C3 fibres) of the cervical plexus to form the ansa cervicalis.

Upper limb

1. **The median nerve**
   a. Commences medial to the axillary artery
   b. Passes deep to flexor digitorum superficialis
   c. Emerges between the palmaris longus and flexor carpi radialis tendons at the wrist
   d. Is supplied by a branch of the posterior interosseous artery
   e. Innervates the wrist joint

2. **The following originate on the radius—**
   a. Flexor pollicis longus
   b. Extensor pollicis longus
   c. Extensor pollicis brevis
   d. Flexor digitorum profundus
   e. Flexor digitorum superficialis

3. **In the upper limb—**
   a. The ulnar nerve passes between the two heads of flexor carpi ulnaris
   b. The musculocutaneous nerve passes between vestiges of the two heads of coracobrachialis
   c. The ulnar artery passes between the two heads of pronator teres
   d. Both heads of biceps are supplied by the same nerve
   e. The heads of the radius and ulna are held together by the annular ligament

4. **At the wrist—**
   a. The ulnar artery is medial to the ulnar nerve
   b. The tendon of abductor pollicis longus hooks around the dorsal tubercle (of Lister)
   c. Palmaris longus is visible in 10% of subjects
   d. Force is transmitted from the hand to the lower end of the ulna
   e. The triquetral articulates with the medial ligament of the wrist joint

Answers overleaf

1. b. c. e.
The medial nerve arises as a medial and a lateral root from the respective brachial plexus cords. The medial root crosses anterior to the axillary artery, hence the median nerve commences lateral to this artery. It usually has no branches in the arm. It passes between the two heads of pronator teres then deep to flexor digitorum superficialis, emerging at the wrist between palmaris longus and the flexor carpi radialis tendons. It is supplied by a branch of the anterior interosseous artery, which was the axial artery of the fetal limb.

2. a. c. e.
The extensor pollicis longus and extensor pollicis brevis originate distal to abductor pollicis longus, with extensor brevis coming off the radius and the adjacent interosseous membrane. The extensor pollicis longus originates on the ulna. Flexor digitorum profundus has a very large origin, which is entirely confined to the ulna and interosseous membrane. Flexor pollicis longus arises from the anterior surface of the radius below the oblique line. Flexor digitorum superficialis has a large origin coming from the medial epicondyle and the medial ligament of the elbow, sublime tubercule of a coronoid process, a fibrous arch between the radius and ulna, as well as the radius itself.

3. a. b. d.
Coracobrachialis is the upper limb's equivalent of the adductor muscles in the thigh. Vestiges of its separate heads can be seen. The musculocutaneous nerve passes between two of these heads. The median nerve passes between the two heads of pronator teres but the ulnar artery is deep to both heads. The musculocutaneous nerve supplies both heads of biceps. The head of the ulna is at its distal end and is therefore not related to the radial head.

4. e.
The ulnar artery is lateral to the ulnar nerve. The tendon of extensor pollicis longus hooks around Lister's tubercle. Palmaris longus is present in 90% of subjects. Force from the hand is transmitted wholly to the distal radius.

5. The radial nerve—
a. Is a direct continuation of the posterior cord of the brachial plexus
b. Contains fibres from the first thoracic spinal nerve
c. Supplies the brachialis muscle
d. Damage in the arm results in a weak grip
e. Has cutaneous branches which cross the anatomical snuff box

6. The anatomical snuff box–
a. Is bounded medially by the extensor pollicis longus tendon
b. Is bounded medially by the extensor pollicis brevis tendon
c. Is bounded laterally by the abductor pollicis longus tendon
d. Has a floor, which is partly formed by the trapezoid bone
e. Contains the cephalic vein, radial artery and the radial nerve

7. The humerus—
a. Has a lesser tuberosity for the insertion of teres minor muscle
b. Forms the lateral margin of the quadrilateral space
c. Has a capitulum, which articulates with the ulnar bone
d. Has a medial epicondyle, which gives rise to the common flexor origin
e. May give rise to the ligament of Struthers

8. The cubital fossa—
a. Contains the brachial artery, which lies lateral to the median nerve
b. Has the brachialis muscle as the lateral boundary
c. Contains the median nerve, which passes between the two heads of flexor carpi ulnaris
d. Contains supratrochlear lymph nodes which receive afferent lymphatic vessels from the third, fourth and fifth fingers and the medial part of the hand and forearm
e. Has the supinator muscle as part of the floor

Answers overleaf

5. All

The fibres from T1 are sensory and are distributed in the posterior cutaneous nerve of the arm. Brachialis is supplied in the main by the musculocutaneous nerve, but is partly supplied by the radial nerve. Damage to the radial nerve in the arm paralyses the finger and wrist extensors causing wrist drop. This position makes the pull of the finger flexors inefficient and results in a weak grip.

6. a. c. e.

The medial boundary of the anatomical snuff box is formed by the extensor pollicis longus tendon. The lateral boundary is formed by the tendons of extensor pollicis brevis and abductor pollicis longus.

The floor is formed by the distal end of the radius, the scaphoid and trapezium bones and the base of the first metacarpal bone.

7. b. d. e.

Subscapularis inserts into the lesser tuberosity.

Teres minor inserts into the lowest of the three facets on the greater tuberosity. The capitulum articulates with the radial head.

The ligament of Struthers is a ligament which attaches to the medial epicondyle of the humerus and to the supracondylar spur of the humerus (if present). The median nerve and/or the brachial artery may pass beneath the ligament of Struthers.

8. a. d. e.

Brachioradialis forms the lateral boundary. Brachialis forms the medial part of the floor.

The median nerve passes between the superficial and deep heads of pronator teres. It is the ulnar nerve which passes between the two heads of flexor carpi ulnaris.

9. **The brachial plexus gives off—**
   a. Suprascapular nerve from the posterior cord
   b. Axillary nerve from the posterior cord, which supplies the deltoid and teres minor muscles
   c. Lateral pectoral nerve from the lateral cord, which supplies pectoralis major and minor muscles
   d. Nerve to subclavius, which may contain fibres to the phrenic nerve
   e. Dorsal scapular nerve from the posterior cord, which supplies levator scapulae, rhomboid major and minor muscles

10. **Structures passing superficial to the flexor retinaculum include—**
    a. Median nerve
    b. Palmaris longus tendon
    c. Palmar cutaneous branch of the ulnar nerve
    d. Palmar cutaneous branch of the radial nerve
    e. Ulnar artery

11. **The axilla—**
    a. Contains the serratus anterior muscle, which forms the medial wall
    b. Contains the biceps brachii and coracobrachialis muscles, which form the lateral wall
    c. Contains the subclavian artery
    d. Contains the long thoracic nerve in the posterior wall
    e. Contains rhomboid major and minor muscles, which form the posterior wall

Answers overleaf

9. b. d.

Suprascapular nerve comes from the upper trunk of the brachial plexus.

Lateral pectoral nerve supplies pectoralis major only.

Dorsal scapular nerve comes from the C5 root of the brachial plexus.

10. b. c. e.

The median nerve passes beneath the flexor retinaculum.

There is no palmar cutaneous branch of the radial nerve. Both the median and ulnar nerves have a palmar cutaneous branch which crosses superficial to the flexor retinaculum.

11. a. b.

The axilla contains the axillary artery, which is a continuation of the subclavian artery at the outer border of the first rib.

The long thoracic nerve lies in the medial wall and supplies the serratus anterior muscle.

Abdomen and pelvis

1. Considering the pancreas—
   a. The neck is anterior to the portal vein
   b. The left suprarenal gland is posterior to the body
   c. The transverse mesocolon is attached to its anterior surface
   d. It receives parasympathetic fibres from the posterior vagal trunk
   e. The head lies at L2

2. The following statements accurately describe the pancreas—
   a. The uncinate process develops as the dorsal pancreatic duct
   b. The accessory pancreatic duct (Santorini) lies posterior to the common bile duct
   c. The head overlies the body of L2 and the aorta
   d. The portal vein lies behind the neck of the pancreas
   e. Endrocrine cells comprise less than 5% of the pancreatic tissue

3. The following structures lie in the transpyloric plane—
   a. The coeliac trunk
   b. The inferior mesenteric artery
   c. The neck of the pancreas
   d. The left kidney
   e. The fundus of the gall bladder

4. In the abdominal wall—
   a. The medial umbilical ligament is a remnant of the urachus
   b. The lateral umbilical ligament passes medial to the deep inguinal ring
   c. The lower part of the rectus abdominis is supplied by the ilioinguinal nerve
   d. The linea alba is wider below than above the umbilicus
   e. The superficial inguinal ring lies lateral to the pubic tubercle

Answers overleaf

1. All

The pancreas is a composite organ having both an exocrine and endocrine function. It lies behind the lesser sac forming most of the bed of the stomach. The transverse mesocolon is attached to its anterior surface just above its inferior margin. Parasympathetic supply, while present, is not essential as the function is predominantly under enteric hormonal control.

2. d. e.

The pancreas develops from dorsal and ventral buds. The ventral becomes the uncinate process. The common bile duct passes posterior to the duct of Santorini.

The neck is that part which lies on the portal vein. The head lies on the inferior vena cava and the body lies partly on the aorta. The endocrine cells comprise 2% of the pancreatic tissue.

3. c. d. e.

The transpyloric plane lies a hand's breadth below the xiphisternum at the level of L1 and the 9th costal cartilage. However, it is strictly defined as the plane half-way between the suprasternal notch and the superior margin of the pubic symphysis. The pancreatic neck, the duodenojejunal flexure and the hila of the kidneys lie in this plane, but the pylorus may not!

4. b.

The *median* umbilical ligament is a remnant of the urachus; the *medial* ligament on each side represents the umbilical artery and the lateral umbilical ligament contains the inferior epigastric vessels. The lateral ligament forms the medial border of the deep inguinal ring. The lower part of rectus is supplied by T12. The linea alba is wider above the umbilicus. An indirect henial sac emerges from the superficial ring medial to the pubic tubercle.

5. Considering the posterior abdominal wall—
   a. The right crus is attached to the bodies of L1 and L2 alone
   b. The subcostal nerve passes beneath the medial arcuate ligament
   c. The iliolumbar artery passes anterior to the psoas major
   d. The femoral nerve emerges lateral to the psoas major
   e. The inferior mesenteric artery arises at L2

6. The diaphragm—
   a. Is derived partly from the dorsal mesentery of the oesophagus
   b. Is supplied with motor fibres from the phrenic and lower intercostal nerves
   c. Its dome rises to the level of the fourth rib in expiration
   d. Is pierced through its left crus by the oesophagus
   e. Interdigitates with the fibres of transversus abdominis

7. Concerning the abdominal aorta—
   a. It is crossed by the left renal vein
   b. Left lumbar veins run posterior to it
   c. Part of the lesser sac lies anteriorly between the origins of the coeliac trunk and superior mesenteric artery
   d. It descends on the vertebral bodies of L1 to L5
   e. It gives a right renal artery which is shorter than the left

8. The portal veir —
   a. Begins behind the head of the pancreas
   b. Runs anterior to the common bile duct
   c. Drains blood from the oesophagus
   d. Lies in the free edge of the greater omentum
   e. Is derived from the vitelline veins

9. The ureter—
   a. Is crossed by the right testicular (ovarian) vein
   b. Is derived from a bud of the paramesonephric duct
   c. Is narrowed at the tip of the transverse process of L3
   d. On the left, is deep to the fourth part of the duodenum
   e. Is crossed by the genitofemoral nerve

Answers overleaf

5. d.
The crura of the diaphragm arise from the bodies of the lumbar vertebrae with the right crus arising from L1–3, and the left crus from L1 and L2. The medial arcuate ligament is a thickening in the fascia over psoas, beneath which passes the sympathetic chain. The lateral arcuate ligament is a thickening in the fascia over quadratus lumborum beneath which the subcostal nerve passes. The iliolumbar artery passes from the pelvis anterior to the lumbosacral trunk but behind psoas major and the obturator nerve. The inferior mesenteric artery arises at L3.

6. a. c. e.
The diaphragm is derived from the dorsal mesentery of the oesophagus, the body wall, the pleuroperitoneal membranes and the septum transversum. Its motor supply is solely from the phrenic nerve. In expiration the dome of the diaphragm rises to the level of the fourth rib anteriorly.

7. a. b. c.
The aorta lies on all the lumbar vertebrae except L5, above which it bifurcates. The right renal artery is longer than the left since it has to travel the diameter of the inferior vena cava to get to the kidney.

8. c. e.
The portal vein begins by the confluence of the splenic and superior mesenteric veins behind the neck of the pancreas. It runs posteromedial to the common bile duct in the free edge of the lesser omentum.

9. a.
Both the testicular (ovarian) vein and the testicular (ovarian) artery cross the ureter. It is derived from a bud of the mesonephric duct. The ureter is narrowed at the pelviureteric junction, the pelvic brim at the level of the sacroiliac joint, and as it pierces the bladder wall. The fourth part of the duodenum does not quite reach the left ureter. The genitofemoral nerve is crossed by the ureter.

10. **The inferior mesenteric artery—**
    a. Crosses the left ureter
    b. Gives off the middle rectal arteries
    c. Has its origin at the level of the third lumbar vertebra
    d. Crosses superficial to the left common iliac artery
    e. Supplies the proximal third of the transverse colon

11. **The inferior vena cava—**
    a. Is related to the right crus of the diaphragm
    b. Is directly anterior to the right adrenal gland
    c. Begins behind the right external iliac artery
    d. Passes through an opening in the central tendon of the diaphragm at the level of T8
    e. Is closely related to the left phrenic nerve

12. **The epiploic foramen—**
    a. Has a superior border formed by the caudate process of the quadrate lobe
    b. Has an inferior border formed by the second part of the duodenum
    c. Has a posterior border formed by the inferior vena cava
    d. Opens into the lesser sac to the left and into Morrison's pouch to the right
    e. Has an anterior border formed by the free right edge of the lesser omentum

13. **The spleen—**
    a. Has a long axis, which lies along the 10th rib
    b. Is connected to the stomach by the gastrosplenic ligament, which contains the left gastroepiploic vessels
    c. Lies on the psoas muscle
    d. Receives its blood supply from a branch of the superior mesenteric artery
    e. When grossly enlarged, may extend across the abdomen towards the right iliac fossa

14. **Derivatives of the midgut include—**
    a. Liver
    b. Pancreas
    c. Meckel's diverticulum
    d. Sigmoid colon
    e. Caecum

Answers overleaf

10. c. d.
The inferior mesenteric artery has its origins at L3 and emerges at the lower border of the third part of the duodenum. It is the artery of the hindgut. It gives off the left colic, sigmoid and superior rectal arteries. The middle rectal arteries are branches of the internal iliac arteries. The main trunk does not cross the left ureter. It usually supplies the distal transverse colon.

11. a. b. d.
The inferior vena cava begins behind the right common iliac artery by the union of the two common iliac veins. It is closely related to the right phrenic nerve.

12. c. d. e.
The superior border is formed by the caudate process of the caudate lobe. The inferior border is formed by the first part of the duodenum.

13. a. b. e.
The splenic artery is a branch of the coeliac axis.
The spleen lies on the 9th, 10th and 11th ribs, and the diaphragm. It does not extend beyond the mid axillary line in normal conditions.

14. c. e.
The liver is derived from the hepatic diverticulum of the foregut and from the septum transversum.
The pancreas is derived from the ventral and dorsal pancreatic buds, which are foregut derivatives. The sigmoid colon is derived from the hindgut.

15. The female bladder—
    a. Has a superior wall, which forms the pouch of Douglas with the uterus
    b. Lies at a lower level than the male counterpart
    c. The anterior wall is related to the pubic symphysis
    d. The apex is connected to the umbilicus
    e. The posterior wall is related to the rectum

16. The anal canal—
    a. Is about 10cm long
    b. Has the voluntary internal anal sphincter formed by the thickening of the circular layer of muscle
    c. In the upper half, contains anal columns of Morgagni
    d. Is derived from the endoderm of the proctadeum in the upper half
    e. Is insensitive to pain

17. The ischiorectal fossa—
    a. Has a lateral boundary formed by the levator ani muscle
    b. Contains the pudendal (Alcock's) canal in its medial wall
    c. Has the external anal sphincter, which forms part of its superomedial wall
    d. Contains the inferior rectal nerve and vessels
    e. Communicates with the opposite fossa in front of and behind the anal canal

Answers overleaf

15. b. d.
The superior wall is covered with peritoneum, which is reflected on to the uterus as the uterovesical pouch. The pouch of Douglas is the pouch formed by the reflection of the peritoneum from the uterus to the rectum (uterorectal pouch).

The bladder lies at a lower level in the female because of the absence of the prostate gland.

There is no anterior wall of the bladder. There are two inferolateral walls which are related to the retropubic pad of fat in the cave of Retzius. The apex of the bladder is connected to the umbilicus via the median umbilical ligament (urachus).

The posterior wall is separated by the cervix and upper vagina from the rectum.

16. c. d.
The anal canal is about 4 cm long.

The internal sphincter is involuntary.

The lower half of the anal canal is sensitive to pain as it is innervated by somatic nerves (inferior rectal branch of the pudendal nerve). The upper half receives autonomic innervation and is therefore insensitive to pain.

17. c. d. e.
The lateral wall of the ischiorectal fossa is formed by the obturator internus covered by the fascia. It has the pudendal canal in its lateral wall.

The superomedial wall is formed by the levator ani muscle and more medially by the external anal sphincter.

Lower limb

1. **Considering the arches of the foot—**
   a. The medial arch is partly supported by bony factors
   b. The spring ligament is important in supporting the medial arch
   c. Peroneus longus tendon predominantly supports the lateral arch
   d. Tibialis posterior has no part in supporting the arches of the foot
   e. The plantar aponeurosis plays a part in supporting the lateral arch

2. **Division of the common peroneal (fibular) nerve causes—**
   a. Anaesthesia of the whole dorsum of the foot
   b. Loss of dorsiflexion of the hallux
   c. Weakness of ankle eversion
   d. Weakness of ankle inversion
   e. Anaesthesia of the lateral side of the little toe

3. **Popliteus—**
   a. Arises from the posterior surface of the tibia below the soleal line
   b. Is attached to the lateral meniscus
   c. Is supplied by the tibial nerve
   d. Is a weak flexor of the knee
   e. Laterally rotates the femur

4. **Considering the relations of the femoral ring—**
   a. The inguinal ligament lies anteriorly
   b. The pectineal ligament lies medially
   c. The femoral artery lies immediately laterally
   d. The superior pubic ramus lies posteriorly
   e. It contains a lymph node draining the female clitoris

Answers overleaf

1. b. c. e.
There are three arches in the foot – medial, longitudinal and lateral. They are supported to varying or no degrees by ligamentous, bony and muscular factors. The medial arch is predominantly supported by ligamentous and muscular attachments, with the shape of the bones providing no support. The plantar aponeurosis helps to support both the medial and lateral arch of the foot whereas peroneus longus tends predominantly to support the lateral arch and has an opposite effect on the medial arch of the foot. Both the tibialis posterior and tibialis anterior help support the medial arch.

2. a. b. c. d.
The common peroneal nerve divides into a deep peroneal and a superficial peroneal nerve. The superficial peroneal nerve supplies the peroneus longus and peroneus brevis muscles which are evertors of the foot. The deep peroneal nerve is the nerve of the extensor compartment of the lower leg and so affects tibialis anterior, extensor digitorum longus and extensor hallucis longus. Inversion usually involves tibialis anterior and tibilais posterior, whereas eversion is predominantly caused by the peroneal muscles. The superficial nerve supplies the whole of the dorsum of the foot except for the first web space. The side of the little toe and most of the lateral side of the foot is supplied by the sural nerve.

3. b. c. e.
Popliteus is a small but important muscle which arises via a fleshy belly from the popliteal surface of the tibia above the soleal line. Its tendon inserts into the lateral femoral condyle but is also attached to the lateral meniscus and helps to move this out of the way in flexion. Its attachment is at the axis of the hinge joint and hence it is not a weak flexor of the knee. It is important for unlocking the knee where it laterally rotates the femur on the tibia.

4. a. e.
The femoral canal which lies within the femoral sheath is widest at its uppermost part, the so-called femoral ring. This is bound by the medial part of the inguinal ligament, posteriorly by the pectineal ligament, medially by the lacunar ligament and laterally by the femoral vein. It contains the lymph node of Cloquet which drains the female clitoris and the male glans penis.

5. In the ankle joint—
   a. The posterior talofibular ligament is attached to the medial tubercle of the talus
   b. The capsule gets its blood supply from the anterior and posterior tibial arteries alone
   c. There is less inversion and eversion in the ankle mortice during plantar flexion
   d. Part of the deltoid ligament is attached to the spring ligament
   e. It is supplied by the deep peroneal nerve

6. The sciatic nerve—
   a. Emerges below piriformis medial to the inferior gluteal nerve and artery
   b. Is in contact with the bone of the ischium
   c. Is crossed superficially by the long head of the rectus femoris
   d. The tibial part may emerge separately by piercing piriformis
   e. Is supplied by a branch of the superior gluteal artery

7. The femoral nerve—
   a. Is derived from the anterior divisions of L2–4
   b. Is contained within the femoral sheath
   c. Has no branches above the inguinal ligament
   d. The nerve to vastus medialis runs in the adductor canal
   e. Supplies sensation to the lateral part of the foot

8. In the lower limb—
   a. Flexor digitorum longus courses superficial to flexor hallucis longus and tibialis posterior
   b. The common fibular (peroneal) nerve can be rolled on the head of the fibula
   c. Fibres of the interosseous membrane slope downwards from tibia to fibula
   d. The peroneal artery runs in the lateral (peroneal) compartment
   e. The bursa under the medial head of gastrocnemius communicates with the synovial cavity of the knee joint

Answers overleaf

5. d. e.
The lateral ligament of the ankle is made up of an anterior and posterior talofibular ligament and the calcaneofibular ligament. The posterior talofibular ligament lies horizontally between the malleolar fossa and the lateral tubercle of the talus. The capsule gets an additional blood supply from the peroneal artery, the talus being wider in front than behind, which means that there is more rocking in plantar flexion than there is in dorsiflexion. The nerve supply is from the deep peroneal nerve as well as the tibial nerve.

6. b.
The sciatic nerve (L4, 5, S1–3) usually emerges as one from below piriformis lateral to the inferior gluteal nerve and vessel. Its two components (tibial and common peroneal) may emerge separately from the pelvis with the common peroneal part percing piriformis. The tibial portion usually emerges from below piriformis. It is crossed by the long head of biceps femoris and is supplied by a branch of the inferior gluteal artery. Because it is in contact with the ischium it may rarely be damaged by posterior dislocations of the hip.

7. d.
The femoral nerve is derived from the posterior division of L2–4 in the lumbar plexus. The obturator nerve is derived from the anterior divisions. The femoral artery, vein and femoral canal are contained within the sheath but not the femoral nerve. There is a branch to the iliacus above the inguinal ligament. The saphenous nerve which runs in the adductor canal supplies the medial side of the foot with sensation.

8. a. c. e.
The new name for the common peroneal nerve is the common fibular nerve. It can still be rolled on the neck of the fibula. The peroneal artery runs in the posterior (flexor) compartment of the leg but supplies the lateral compartment by its branches. The bursa under the medial head of gastrocnemius always communicates with the knee joint but only sometimes with the semimembranosus bursa.

9. **In the groin—**
   a. The femoral nerve lies in the lateral part of the femoral sheath
   b. The femoral branch of the genitofemoral nerve pierces the femoral sheath
   c. The pubic tubercle is located by following adductor magnus to its origin
   d. Scarpa's fascia attaches to the lower edge of the inguinal ligament
   e. The lymph node of Cloquet is said to drain directly from the glans penis

10. **At the hip joint—**
    a. Psoas acts as a medial rotator of the thigh
    b. Acetabulum means a deep depression
    c. The capsule extends anteriorly along the neck to the trochanteric line
    d. The iliofemoral ligament is attached to the anterior superior iliac spine
    e. The femoral head is supplied by branches of the trochanteric anastomosis

11. **In the region of the ankle—**
    a. The great saphenous vein lies in front of the lateral malleolus
    b. The tendon of peroneus longus grooves the malleolar fossa
    c. The distal tibiofibular joint is synovial
    d. Flexor hallucis longus is found between the tubercles of the posterior process of the talus
    e. Tibialis posterior passes below the sustentaculum tali

12. **The popliteal fossa—**
    a. Is bounded superolaterally by the semimembranosus and semitendinosus muscles
    b. Has the popliteus muscle as part of its floor
    c. Contains the posterior cutaneous nerve of the thigh in its roof
    d. Contains the superficial peroneal nerve
    e. Has the popliteal artery, which lies deeper than the tibial nerve

Answers overleaf

9. a. e.
The femoral nerve is lateral to but not within the femoral sheath.
Following the tendon of adductor longus proximally leads to the
pubic tubercle. Scarpa's fascia (the fibrous part of the superficial
fascia) attaches to the fascia lata at the flexure skin crease of the hip
joint. This attachment is the lower limit of the space into which
urine can extravasate when the urethra ruptures.

10. a. c. e.
Acetabulum means a vinegar cup! Posteriorly the capsule extends
halfway along the neck, but anteriorly it passes to the trochanteric
line. The iliofemoral ligament (of Bigelow) is attached above to the
anterior inferior iliac spine. The retinacular vessels are derived from
the trochanteric anastomosis and go to supply the femoral head.
The precise action of psoas is not clear, but a full discussion of it
can be found in *Gray's Anatomy*.

11. d.
The great saphenous vein is anterior to the medial malleolus. It is
peroneus brevis which grooves the malleolar fossa. The skull
sutures and distal tibiofibular joints are the only fibrous joints of
the body. Flexor hallucis longus hooks under the sustentaculum.

12. b. c. e.
The superolateral boundary is formed by the biceps femroris
muscle. The semimembranosus and semitendinosus muscles form
the superomedial boundary. The fossa contains the common
peroneal nerve. The superficial peroneal nerve is one of the two
terminal brances of the common peroneal nerve and it arises in the
substance of the peroneus longus muscle.

Thorax

1. **The following muscles have attachments to costal cartilages—**
   a. Pectoralis major
   b. Diaphragm
   c. External oblique
   d. Iliocostalis
   e. Transversus abdominis

2. **Concerning the first rib—**
   a. The head has a single articular facet
   b. Scalenus medius attaches to the scalene tubercle
   c. The supreme intercostal vein lies medial to the superior intercostal artery
   d. It is in close contact with the T1 nerve root
   e. The costoclavicular ligament attaches to its sternal end

3. **The sternal angle (angle of Louis)—**
   a. Marks the demarcation between the superior and the inferior mediastinum
   b. Marks the level of the top of the aortic arch
   c. Corresponds to the level of the intervertebral disc between the third and fourth thoracic vertebrae
   d. Marks the level of the second costal cartilage
   e. Marks the level where the azygous vein drains into the superior vena cava

4. **In the thorax—**
   a. The azygous vein is formed by the right subcostal vein and first and second lumbar veins
   b. The right coronary artery arises from the right posterior sinus of the aorta
   c. The right subclavian artery may arise directly from the aortic arch
   d. Both common carotids are derived from the third branchial arch
   e. The external intercostal muscle forms the posterior intercostal membrane at the angle of the ribs

Answers overleaf

1. a. b. e.
Pectoralis major is attached to the upper six costal cartilages. The diaphragm and transversus abdominis interdigitate at their attachments to the costal cartilages at the costal margin. Iliocostalis is part of the erector spinae group and attaches to the angles of the lower six ribs.

2. a. c. d. e.
The first rib is an atypical rib in which there is a single articular facet. The sympathetic chain runs most medially across the neck with the supreme intercostal vein and superior intercostal artery more laterally respectively. Scalenus anterior attaches to the scalene tubercle with scalenus medius attaching to a smoother area of superior surface of the shaft.

3. a. d. e.
The sternal angle marks the beginning and the end of the aortic arch, not the top of the aortic arch. The entire aortic arch lies behind the manubrium sterni in the superior mediastinum.

The sternal angle corresponds to the level of the intervertebral disc between the fourth and the fifth thoracic vertebrae.

4. a. c. d.
The right coronary artery arises from the anterior aortic sinus whereas the left coronary artery arises from the left posterior aortic sinus. The right subclavian may arise from the aortic arch and in passing behind the oesophagus may well constrict it, a condition called dysphagia lusoria. The external intercostal muscle extends from the superior costotransverse ligament posteriorly, to the costochondral junction anteriorly, where it becomes the anterior intercostal membrane. The internal intercostal muscle extends from the side of the sternum to the angle of the rib, where it becomes a posterior intercostal membrane.

5. **The oesophagus—**
   a. Is partly supplied by branches of the inferior thyroid artery
   b. Is about 25 cm long
   c. Is overlapped by the bifurcation of the trachea
   d. Has a constriction at the level of C6
   e. Passes through the diaphragm together with the two vagi at the level of T10

6. **The diaphragm—**
   a. Is partly derived from the dorsal mesentery
   b. Has a right crus which is bigger than the left
   c. Has an opening in its central tendon for the passage of inferior vena cava at the level of T8 together with the left phrenic nerve
   d. Has motor innervation from the phrenic and lower intercostal nerves
   e. Has sensory innervation from the lower intercostal nerves

7. **The venous drainage of the heart includes—**
   a. The great cardiac vein, which runs in the posterior interventricular groove
   b. The coronary sinus, which is the continuation of the great cardiac vein
   c. The small cardiac vein, which drains into the coronary sinus
   d. The Thebesian veins (venae cordis minimae), which drain into the coronary sinus
   e. The oblique vein of the left atrium, which drains into the coronary sinus

8. **The azygous vein—**
   a. Represents the persistent right posterior cardinal vein of the embryo
   b. Receives the right first (supreme) intercostal vein
   c. Arches over the right main bronchus at T4
   d. Runs anterior to the right intercostal arteries
   e. Drains blood from the hemiazygous vein

Answers overleaf

5. a. b. d. e.
The oesophagus is overlapped by the left main bronchus, not by the bifurcation of the trachea.

6. a. b. e.
The inferior vena cava passes through the central tendon of the diaphragm together with the right phrenic nerve at the level of T8.

Motor innervation of the diaphragm comes from the phrenic nerves only.

7. b. c. e.
The great cardiac vein runs in the anterior interventricular groove.

The Thebesian veins (venae cordis minimae) drain directly into the chambers of the heart.

8. a. c. d. e.
The supreme intercostal vein drains into the vertebral vein or brachiocephalic vein on each side. The right intercostal arteries run posterior to the azygous vein and the left intercostal veins run posterior to the aorta (except the supreme and superior intercostal veins). The hemiazygous and accessory hemiazygous veins drain into the azygous vein by a channel or channels passing to the right posterior to the thoracic duct.

9. **The aorta—**
   a. Passes through the diaphragm at the level of T10
   b. Is crossed by the left phrenic nerve and left vagus nerve
   c. Has an arch, which commences and ends at the angle of Louis
   d. Supplies the proximal third of the oesophagus
   e. Lies anterior to the trachea in the superior mediastinum

10. **The following veins usually drain into the left brachiocephalic vein—**
    a. Vertebral
    b. Thymic
    c. Internal thoracic
    d. Inferior thyroid
    e. Left supreme intercostal vein

11. **In a full-term baby—**
    a. The left brachiocephalic vein may lie above the level of the sternal notch
    b. The distal femoral epiphysis is visible on X-ray
    c. The metopic suture could be mistaken for a fracture of the parietal bone
    d. The mastoid process covers the emerging facial nerve
    e. The inferior border of the liver is palpable below the costal margin

12. **In the fetus—**
    a. The ductus arteriosus is derived from the left fifth aortic arch artery
    b. The left umbilical vein carries oxgenated blood
    c. Oxygenated blood bypasses the liver via the ductus arteriosus
    d. The closure of the foramen ovale at birth is due to increased left atrial pressure
    e. The third arch artery contributes to the common carotid artery

Answers overleaf

9. b. c. e.
The aorta passes through the diaphragm at the level of T12. It is the oesophagus which pierces the diaphragm at the level of T10.

The aorta generally supplies the middle third of the oesophagus; the promixal third is usually supplied by branches of the inferior thyroid artery.

10. All
The superior intercostal veins and thoracic duct also drain into the left brachiocephalic vein.

11. a. b. e.
Care must be taken in performing a tracheostomy on a baby because the left brachiocephalic vein often lies above the sternal notch. The distal epiphysis of the femur is ossified at birth. The metopic suture lies in the midline between the frontal bones. It usually fuses by 6 years of age but may persist. It may be mistaken for a fracture of the frontal bone but surely not the parietal bone. The mastoid process is rudimentary in the neonate and the facial nerve is thus relatively exposed to trauma, e.g. by forceps delivery.

12. b. d. e.
The ductus arteriosus is derived from the left sixth aortic arch artery. It connects the aortic arch with the pulmonary trunk. The fifth aortic arch disappears.

Oxygenated blood from the placenta is carried in the left umbilical vein. It bypasses the liver via the ductus venosus.

13. The following statement(s) is/are true—
 a. The suprasternal notch lies at the level of the second thoracic vertebra
 b. The femoral pulse is found at the midpoint between the anterior superior iliac spine and the pubic tubercle
 c. The dorsalis pedis pulse is found in front of the ankle joint between the tibialis anterior tendon and the extensor hallucis longus tendon
 d. The root of the spine of the scapula lies at the level of the third thoracic vertebra
 e. The iliac crest lies at the level of the fourth lumbar vertebra

Answers overleaf

13. a. d. e.

The femoral pulse is found at the midpoint between the anterior superior iliac spine and the symphysis pubis.

The dorsalis pedis pulse is found in front of the ankle joint between the extensor hallucis longus tendon and the extensor digitorum longus tendon.

Physiology MCQs

Nerve and muscle

1. At a neuromuscular junction in biceps femoris—
   a. The terminal knobs are unmyelinated
   b. Several nerve fibres impinge on each endplate
   c. The miniature endplate potentials are caused by quantal release of noradrenaline
   d. The synapses are made en passant
   e. Calcium ions are required for transmitter release

2. At a sympathetic postganglionic ending—
   a. Clear presynaptic vesicles contain noradrenaline
   b. Reuptake of noradrenaline is mostly passive
   c. Monoamine oxidase is located mainly in the presynaptic cell
   d. Presynaptic alpha$_2$ receptors inhibit further release of transmitter
   e. Dopamine is a precursor in the synthesis of noradrenaline

3. In human skeletal muscle—
   a. The A band corresponds to lines of thin filaments
   b. During contraction the width of the A band decreases
   c. Tetanic contraction produces four times the tension of a single twitch
   d. The resting membrane potential is about –90 mV
   e. The T tubule system acts as a store of calcium

4. Considering a myelinated nerve—
   a. The action potential is conducted in both directions along the axon
   b. Conduction velocity is proportional to the square of the radius
   c. Repolarization relies partly on a decrease in potassium permeability
   d. Excitability of the nerve is increased by raised extracellular calcium levels
   e. The spike potential lasts 50 ms

Answers overleaf

1. a. e.
One nerve fibre impinges on each endplate. Synapses en passant are found in smooth muscle. The miniature endplate potentials are caused by quantal release of acetylcholine. Arrival of an action potential at the nerve terminal increases the calcium permeability which is responsible for transmitter release.

2. c. d. e.
Noradrenaline is found in dense core vesicles; acetylcholine is found in clear vesicles. The process of reuptake is active. Dopamine is the immediate precursor of noradrenaline in the synthetic pathway.

3. c. d.
The A band corresponds to lines of thick filaments and does not shorter during contraction. The T tubules help transmission of the action potential to muscle fibrils. It is the terminal cisterns of the sarcoplasmic reticulum which store calcium.

4. a.
Conduction velocity in myelinated nerves is proportional to the diameter. In unmyelinated nerves it is proportional to the square root of the diameter. Repolarization relies on an increase in K permeability. High extracellular calcium stabilizes the membrane by decreasing its excitability. The spike lasts 0.5–1 ms in a myelinated nerve.

5. **Muscle spindles—**
   a. Are innervated by groups Ib and II afferents
   b. Are extrafusal fibres
   c. Record the tension developed in the muscle
   d. Receive motor innervation from gamma fibres, which are myelinated
   e. Play an important role in maintaining muscle tone

6. **In the control of muscle contraction—**
   a. Tropomyosin is a globular protein
   b. Actin binds to myosin in the absence of calcium ions when troponins and tropomyosin are removed
   c. Troponin C binds to calcium
   d. Troponin and tropomyosin are important in striated muscle not smooth muscle
   e. Troponin masks the myosin-combining sites on the actin

7. **The conduction velocity of nerve fibres is increased by—**
   a. Increasing temperature
   b. Decreasing temperature
   c. Increasing external ionic sodium concentration
   d. Decreasing external ionic sodium concentration
   e. Decreasing axon diameter

8. **Nerve fibres—**
   a. Of the A-beta type are responsible for the transmission of touch and pressure modalities
   b. Transmitting pain and temperature modalities are carried by the A-delta and C fibres
   c. Of A-delta type are myelinated
   d. Of the A-alpha type conduct at a velocity of between 30 and 50 m/s
   e. Conduct faster if myelinated

9. **Substances which decrease the release of acetylcholine from presynaptic cholinergic nerve terminals include—**
   a. Atropine
   b. Botulinum toxin
   c. Amitriptyline
   d. Hemicholinium-3
   e. Reserpine

Answers overleaf

5. d. e.
Muscle spindles receive their sensory innervation from Ia and II fibres.

The Ib fibres supply the Golgi tendon organs.

Muscle spindles are known as intrafusal fibres whereas the normal muscle fibres themselves are known as extrafusal fibres.

They record length (static) and rate of change in length (dynamic), not tension.

6. b. c. d.
Tropomyosin consists of two polypeptide chains located in the groove formed by the actin filaments. Troponins consists of three globular proteins located on every seventh actin monomer.

It is the tropomyosin which masks the myosin-combining sites on the actin.

7. a. c.
The conduction velocity is increased by increasing temperature, increasing axonal diameter, increasing ionic sodium concentration and myelination of nerve fibre.

0. a. b. c. c.
A-alpha fibres conduct at a velocity of between 70 and 120 m/s.

Conduction velocity increases with myelination of fibre, increasing temperature, increasing axonal diameter and increasing ionic sodium concentration.

9. b. d.
Atropine is a competitive antagonist at the receptor site. It does not decrease the release of acetylcholine.

Amitriptyline is an uptake inhibitor at the presynaptic noradrenergic and 5-hydroxytriptaminergic neurons.

Reserpine depletes noradrenaline from the nerve terminals.

Central nervous system

1. **Cerebrospinal fluid—**
   a. Is produced at a rate of approximately 750 ml/day
   b. Is predominantly secreted by the choroid plexus in the lateral ventricles
   c. Has a similar specific gravity to that of the brain
   d. Has a higher potassium concentration compared to plasma
   e. Pressure increases in haemorrhage and infection

2. **The following are neurotransmitters—**
   a. Dihydroxyphenylalanine
   b. Dipalmitoylphosphatidylcholine
   c. Glycine
   d. Leu-enkephalin
   e. Somatostatin

3. **The pattern of the electroencephalogram may be altered in the following conditions—**
   a. Hypoglycaemia
   b. Portosystemic encephalopathy
   c. Hypothermia
   d. Cerebral tumours
   e. Sympathetic discharge

4. **The pH of the cerebrospinal fluid—**
   a. Fluctuates more rapidly than that of the plasma
   b. Is decreased more rapidly by lactic acid than by carbon dioxide
   c. Is normally higher than the arterial pH
   d. Is detected by medullary chemoreceptors
   e. Falls in the acute phase of acclimatization to high altitude

5. **The hypothalamus—**
   a. Contains thermoreceptors, which detect the core temperature
   b. Secretes antidiuretic hormone into the portal hypophyseal vessels
   c. Secretes a prolactin-releasing factor, which may be dopamine
   d. Synthesizes oxytocin and vasopressin in the supraoptic and paraventricular nuclei
   e. Contains suprachiasmatic nuclei, which receive inputs from the retina

Answers overleaf

1. a. b. c. e.
The volume of cerebrospinal fluid in humans is approximately 150 ml at any one time. It is produced at a rate of 600–750 ml/day. Up to 70% is secreted by the choroid plexus in all four ventricles but mainly in the lateral ventricles. It is also secreted by ependymal surfaces. The fact that cerebrospinal fluid has a similar specific gravity to that of the brain means that the brain can float, thus it is supported within the cranial cavity. The potassium concentration is lower than in the plasma. There is an increase in cerebrospinal fluid pressure in haemorrhage and infection, as there are an increased number of cells leading to blockage of absorption channels.

2. a. c. d. e.
Dihyroxyphenylalanine is dopamine. Dipalmitoylphosphatidylcholine is a constituent of surfactant. Somatostatin is a probable transmitter at the dorsal horn of the spinal cord.

3. All
At rest, in an unstimulated subject, the alpha rhythm (10 Hz) is seen. The frequency decreases in hypoglycaemia, low cortisol, hypothermia and raised arterial P_{CO_2}. Tumours cause the development of irregular slow waves and sympathetic discharge activates the reticular activating system.

4. a. d.
The pH of the cerebrospinal fluid changes more rapidly than the arterial pH because the former contains very little protein, which means it has a lower buffering capacity.
    Lactic acid cannot diffuse through the blood–brain barrier, whereas carbon dioxide can.
    The pH of the cerebrospinal fluid rises in the acute phase of acclimatization to high altitude due to hyperventilation.

5. a. d. e.
Antidiuretic hormone is synthesized by neurons of the supraoptic and paraventricular nuclei and is released in the posterior pituitary lobe via the hypothalamohypophyseal tract.
    The protlactin-inhibiting factor is probably dopamine. The releasing factor is unknown, but thyrotropin-releasing hormone and vasoactive intestinal peptide are known to increase its secretion.

6. The retina—

a. Contains about 125 million rods

b. Contains only cones at the fovea centralis

c. Has cones containing red-sensitive, blue-sensitive and yellow-sensitive pigments

d. Contains horizontal and amacrine cells which are important in lateral inhibition

e. Contains rhodopsin which changes to the *cis*-form on exposure to light

Answers overleaf

6. a. b. d.

The retina contains green-sensitive not yellow-sensitive pigments.

The rhodopsin molecule changes from the *cis*-form to the *trans*-form on exposure to light.

Cardiorespiratory

1. **Concerning the Valsalva manoeuvre—**
   a. It is highly dependent on baroreceptor activity
   b. Secondary hyperaldosteronism disrupts the heart rate and blood pressure changes when intrathoracic pressure returns to normal
   c. There is a brief fall in blood pressure at the onset of straining
   d. It is of value to the anaesthetist in assessment of autonomic function
   e. Its response is diminished in the presence of hypovolaemia

2. **The following circulatory changes occur in the newborn—**
   a. Peripheral vascular resistance decreases
   b. Left atrial pressure increases
   c. Pulmonary vascular resistance increases
   d. The ductus arteriosus closes within 4–6 hours
   e. The right and left heart change from pumping in series to pumping in parallel

3. **During the normal cardiac cycle—**
   a. The majority of ventricular filling occurs as a result of atrial systole
   b. The normal ejection fraction is about 65%
   c. The a-wave of the jugular venous pulse is due to tricuspid bulging during ventricular systole
   d. The interventricular septum depolarizes from right to left
   e. Pacemaker activity is situated near to the junction of the right atrium and inferior vena cava

Answers overleaf

1. a. d. e.
The Valsalva manoeuvre is forced expiration against a closed glottis and is dependent on functioning baroreceptor activity. At the onset of straining the blood pressure rises as the increased intrathoracic pressure adds to the pressure of blood in the aorta. The blood pressure then decreases as the raised intrathoracic pressure decreases venous return by pressing the intrathoracic veins. This decease in pressure stimulates the baroreceptors, which leads to a tachycardia and a rise in peripheral resistance. Once the glottis is open there is an initial increase in blood pressure as the cardiac output returns to normal but it is functioning against the raised peripheral resistance. The sympathetomized patient's heart rate changes still occur but are absent in autonomic insufficiency such as occurs in diabetes mellitus. The response is diminished during hypovolaemia due to the fact that the patient has increased sympathetic activity. Primary hyperaldosteronism for reasons unknown disrupts the Valsalva manoeuvre.

2. b.
After birth the placental circulation is cut off, so increasing peripheral vascular resistance. As a result of this loss of placental function, the infant becomes increasingly hypoxic. Under the influence of this and other external stimuli it inspires for the first time. This decreases pulmonary vascular resistance so increasing left atrial return, with the result of the increase in left atrial pressure. Ductus arteriosus first narrows and then usually closes completely within 2 days. In the fetal circulation, the right and left hearts are pumping in parallel and change to be in series after birth.

3. b.
Initial cardiac depolarization occurs at the sinoatrial node which is situated in the right atrium near its junction with the superior vena cava. The conducting system transmitting impulses from here depolarizes the interventricular septum from left to right. The a-wave of the jugular venous pulse corresponds to atrial systole whereas the c-wave is transmitted as a result of tricuspid bulging during ventricular systole. The majority of ventricular filling occurs passively with a maximum of approximately 30% occurring as a result of atrial systole. The end-diastolic ventricular volume is 130 ml of blood with each normal stroke ejecting 70–90 ml of blood from each venticle, thus the ejection fraction is 65%.

4. Considering the venous system
a. In a perfectly still, upright person, venous pressure in the foot is about 90 mmHg
b. In a healthy walking subject, venous pressure in the foot is about 125 mmHg
c. Central venous pressure in a healthy subject is about 0 mmHg
d. Central venous pressure falls greatly in cardiac tamponade
e. Pressure in the sagittal sinus may be subatmospheric

5. Concerning the circulation—
a. Mean arterial pressure is 120 mmHg in a 30-year-old man
b. A collapsing pulse is found in persistent ductus arteriosus
c. Blood viscosity is determined primarily by the concentration of plasma proteins
d. An increase in total peripheral resistance results in an increase in pulse pressure
e. Some 65% of blood volume resides in the veins

6. In carbon monoxide poisoning—
a. The gas forms carbamino compounds with haemoglobin
b. The resultant hypoxia causes stimulation of carotid chemoreceptors
c. There is a decrease in haemoglobin concentration
d. Ventilation with fresh air is a better treatment than ventilation with oxygen
e. Treatment with hyperbaric oxygen may be indicated

7. The following statements are true of the tetralogy of Fallot—
a. There is a left-to-right shunt
b. Right ventricular pressure is raised
c. There is an atrial septal defect
d. The amount of deoxygenated haemoglobin in arterial blood may be over 5 g/dl
e. The affected children squat to decrease the amount of shunting

Answers overleaf

4. a. c. e.
When walking, the muscle pump and competent venous valves help to decrease venous pooling and the pressure in the foot falls to about 25 mmHg. Normal central venous pressure varies around 0 mmHg. In cardiac tamponade the central venous pressure rises due to an increased resistance to venous return causing a damming-up of blood. The dural sinuses are unable to collapse because their walls are held apart by their attachments. Therefore on standing, pressure inside the sinuses becomes subatmospheric.

5. b. e.
Mean arterial pressure is usually between 90 and 100 mmHg in a fit 30-year-old male. A collapsing pulse is found in aortic regurgitation and persistent ductus arteriosus. Blood viscosity is determined primarily by the concentration of red blood cells. Changes in total peripheral resistance cause the pulse pressure to change in the opposite direction.

6. e.
Carbamino compounds are formed by carbon dioxide whereas carbon monoxide forms carbonmonoxyhaemoglobin (carboxyhaemoglobin). The PO_2 is unchanged so there will not be stimulation of chemoreceptors. The haemoglobin concentration is also unchanged. Oxygen hastens the dissociation of carboxyhaemoglobin so oxygen is preferable to fresh air. Hyperbaric oxygen is available in specialist centres and may be indicated in the treatment of carbon monoxide poisoning.

7. b. d. e.
The tetralogy consists of a ventricular septal defect, and aorta overriding both ventricles and the ventricular septal defect, pulmonary tract stenosis and right ventricular hypertrophy. It accounts for 10% of cases of congenital heart disease. Cyanosis is common. Squatting raises the resistance to left ventricular ejection and therefore decreases the degree of right-to-left shunt.

8. Turbulent flow of blood tends to occur—
 a. When the viscosity of the blood is increased
 b. When the radius of the vessel is increased
 c. When the velocity of blood flow is decreased
 d. At much lower flow velocities with steady flow than with pulsatile flow
 e. Commonly in the normal circulation

9. Haemoglobin—
 a. Has a molecular weight of approximately 65 000 Da
 b. Has a substitution at the beta-6 position (where glutamic acid is replaced by valine) in sickle cell anaemia
 c. When combined with carbon monoxide is called carboxy-haemoglobin
 d. In the adult, contains less 2,3-DPG than in the fetus
 e. In the fetus contains two alpha subunits and two delta subunits

10. The resistance to blood flow—
 a. Increases with increasing viscosity of the blood
 b. Increases with decreasing length of the vessel
 c. Is proportional to the fourth root of the radius
 d. Is inversely proportional to the fourth power of the radius
 e. Is inversely proportional to the blood flow

11. The oxygen dissociation curve—
 a. Is shifted to the right by 2,3-DPG
 b. Is sigmoid shape for both haemoglobin and myoglobin
 c. Is shifted to the left when one ascends to high altitude
 d. Is shifted to the right by an increase in the pH
 e. Is ideally 50% saturated at a PO_2 of 28 mmHg.

12. During exercise—
 a. Pulmonary ventilation increases up to a maximum of 10-fold
 b. The depth of ventilation increases before the rate
 c. Oxygen debt can occur up to a maximum of 20 litres
 d. The total peripheral resistance falls
 e. Energy is derived from the local glycogen store rather than from extra muscular carbohydrate

Answers overleaf

8. b. d.
Probability of turbulence increases as $\dfrac{\text{radius of vessel} \times \text{velocity of flow}}{\text{viscosity}}$ increases.

Therefore, turbulent blood flow occurs with increasing radius and flow velocity and decreasing viscosity.

Turbulent blood flow is uncommon in the normal circulation because flow is pulsatile.

9. a. b. c.
Fetal haemoglobin contains two alpha and two gamma subunits. Haemoglobin containing two alpha and two delta subunits is called HbA2.

When haemoglobin is combined with carbon dioxide it is called carbamino compound. Fetal haemoglobin contains less 2,3-DPG than adult haemoglobin, which explains the fact that the fetal oxygen dissociation curve is to the left of that for the adult. Hence fetal haemoglobin has a higher affinity for oxygen than adult haemoglobin and is able to extract oxygen from maternal haemoglobin in the placenta.

10. a. d. e.
The resistance is proportional to $\dfrac{\text{length of vessel} \times \text{viscosity}}{\text{radius}^4}$

$$\text{Blood flow} = \frac{\text{driving force}}{\text{resistance to flow}}$$

11. a. e.
The curve for myoglobin is a rectangular hyperbola as it only binds 1 rather than 4 moles of oxygen per mole of myoglobin.

The haemoglobin curve is shifted to the right by an increase in 2,3-DPG, a decrease in pH, an increase in $P\text{CO}_2$, and an increase in the temperature. At high altitude, the curve is shifted to the right due to an increase in 2,3-DPG, in order to unload oxygen to the tissues.

12. b. c. d. e.
Pulmonary ventilation can increase up to 30-fold (from 5 l to 150 l/min).

In mild exercise, the depth of ventilation increases. In moderate to severe exercise, the depth and the rate of ventilation increase.

The total peripheral resistance falls in exercise in order to allow an increase in the cardiac output.

13. On ascent to high altitude—
   a. There is increased erythropoietin secretion
   b. Mountain sickness is mainly caused by cerebral oedema
   c. The cardiac output is reduced
   d. The oxygen dissociation curve is shifted to the right
   e. Pulmonary oedema can occur in the unacclimatized individual

14. Cardiac muscle—
   a. Is essentially non-syncytial
   b. Has an action potential lasting about 250 ms
   c. Cannot be tetanized because the action potential is nearly half over when contraction begins
   d. Relies on a delayed decrease in calcium permeability for its action potential plateau
   e. At rest, derives 60% of its energy requirement from fat

Answers overleaf

13. a. b. d. e.
On ascent to high altitude, the cardiac output is increased to provide more oxygen to the tissues.

The oxygen dissociation curve is shifted to the right due to an increase in 2,3-DPG, which has the effect of increased delivery of oxygen to the tissues.

14. b. e.
Cardiac muscle cannot be tetanized because the action potential has a long absolute refractory period and contraction is nearly half over by the time a second action potential can be initiated.

The plateau depends on an increase in calcium permeability. At rest 60% of cardiac muscle energy is derived from fat, 35% from carbohydrate and 5% from ketones.

Renal

1. **In considering normal renal physiology—**
   a. Glomerular filtration pressure is of the order of 10 mmHg
   b. The filtration fraction is approximately 20%
   c. Some red blood cells are usually found in the glomerular filtrate
   d. The majority of the blood supply is to the medulla
   e. Inulin is neither secreted nor reabsorbed

2. **Concerning renal volume excretion—**
   a. An increase in the glomerular filtration rate of 50% can increase urine output by approximately 10-fold
   b. It is governed acutely by the presence of osmotic diuretics
   c. Average urine volume excretion is 2.5 1/24 h
   d. Arterial blood pressure has an important long-term effect
   e. An increased plasma oncotic pressure increases both the glomerular filtration pressure and tubular reabsorption

Answers overleaf

1. a. b. e.
The glomerular filtration pressure is equal to the hydrostatic pressure in the glomerulus, minus the sum of the hydrostatic pressure in the Bowman's capsule and the oncotic pressure in the glomerulus. This usually amounts to approximately 10 mmHg. The filtration fraction is the proportion of the glomerular filtration rate compared to the renal plasma flow. Glomerular filtration is usually 125 ml/min whereas the normal renal plasma flow is 650 ml/min. Red blood cells do not usually cross the functional structure of the glomerular membrane. The majority of the blood supply is to the cortex where the glomeruli are situated. Inulin is a polysaccharide that is small enough to pass through the glomerulus membrane but which is not significantly reabsorbed; therefore it is only filtered and is used to measure glomerular filtration rate.

2. a. b. d.
Average urine volume excretion is normally 1.5 l/day. This is governed by the balance between the glomerular filtration rate and tubular reabsorption. Under normal conditions, nearly the whole of the glomerular filtrate is reabsorbed, although this is never 100%. As the glomerular filtration rate increases there is an increasing discrepancy, such that there is an increasing difference between the glomerular filtration rate and the amount of fluid reabsorbed; thus a small change in the glomerular filtration rate may lead to large changes in urine output. Movement of fluid within the glomerular tubles is governed mainly by Starling's law governing movement of fluid in capillaries. Thus the glomerular filtration pressure is equal to the glomerular pressure minus the sum of the glomerular osmotic pressure and capsular pressure. An increased plasma oncotic pressure decreases glomerular filtration pressure whereas it increases tubular reabsorption. Glomerular blood pressure is perhaps the most important factor in governing urine output as it increases the glomerular filtration pressure and decreases reabsorption. The osmotic diuretics prevent reabsorption of water and hence increase urine output.

3. Renal autoregulation—
   a. Is important in maintaining renal blood flow in renal artery stenosis
   b. Acts mainly between a blood pressure of 70–160 mmHg
   c. Is thought to be highly dependent on the sodium concentration of the glomerular filtrate at the macula densa
   d. May autoregulate renal blood flow through efferent arteriolar vasoconstriction
   e. Is important in helping to maintain urea excretion during hypotensive episodes

4. Concerning the ureter—
   a. Peristalsis relies on the presence of an intact extrinsic innervation
   b. Ureteral activity decreases as renal urine output decreases
   c. Obstruction by a stone causes reflex bradycardia and sweating
   d. Ureterocolic anastomosis leads to oliguria in the early postoperative period
   e. Ureterosigmoidostomy predisposes to hypochloraemic acidosis

5. Renin—
   a. Is secreted by the cells of the macula densa
   b. Secretion is decreased by prostaglandins
   c. Is a decapeptide
   d. Acts to form a potent vasoconstrictor from angiotensin I
   e. Levels are raised in the standing subject

6. In renal tubular function—
   a. Amino acids are reabsorbed in the proximal convoluted tubules by a single carrier mechanism
   b. Distal convoluted tubules contain columnar cells with a brush border
   c. Sodium reabsorption is associated with isosmotic water reabsorption in the distal convoluted tubules
   d. Phosphate reabsorption is decreased by parathyroid hormone
   e. The transverse gradient of the countercurrent system is caused by an active secretion of sodium ions from the thick ascending limb

Answers overleaf

3. b. e.
Renal autoregulation is involved in regulating the glomerular filtration rate as well as the renal blood flow, to maintain them within normal limits while blood pressure varies. Its main range of action is between 75 and 160 mmHg. The process of autoregulation involves an afferent arteriolar vasodilator feedback mechanism as well as an efferent arteriolar vasoconstrictor feedback mechanism, both of which are dependent on the concentration of chloride ions at the macula densa. Blood flow is only autoregulated in the early stages of blood pressure change via the afferent vasodilator mechanism. The efferent arteriolar vasoconstrictor mechanism becomes more potent as the blood pressure change continues and is principally involved with the maintenance of the glomerular filtration rate; thus during hypotensive episodes the glomerular filtration rate is maintained so that urea may be excreted. As renal artery stenosis is a chronic disease there is very little autoregulation of the blood flow.

4. b. d.
Peristalsis of the ureter does not rely on the presence of extrinsic innervation but its activity is proportional to the volume flow of urine. The response to ureteral obstruction is reflex tachycardia and sweating. Oliguria after ureterocolic anastomosis may be caused by oedema of the anastomosis site. Metabolic changes after ureterosigmoidostomy usually consist of a hyperchloraemic acidosis.

5. e.
Renin is secreted by cells of the juxtaglomerular apparatus and is a glycoprotein of molecular weight 40 000. Renin forms angiotensin I from angiotensinogen.

6. d. e.
Amino acids are reabsorbed by four carrier mechanisms – acidic, basic, neutral and imino acid mechanisms in the proximal convoluted tubules.

Isosmotic water reabsorption occurs in the proximal convoluted tubules. The transverse current is now thought to be caused by an active secretion of sodium ions (rather than chloride ions) from the thick ascending limb of the loop of Henle.

Endocrine

1. The following are true of insulin—
  a. It is a polypeptide composed of two amino acid chains
  b. Its secretion is affected by glucagon
  c. It stimulates gluconeogenesis
  d. It has little or no effect on the uptake of glucose in the brain
  e. If lacking it may be a cause of a fatty liver

2. Regarding the breast—
  a. Oestrogens are primarily responsible for the development of ducts
  b. Full lobuloalveolar development is completed at puberty
  c. Milk is secreted into the ducts as early as the fifth month of pregnancy
  d. Prolactin causes contraction of the myoepithelial cells
  e. Human milk contains more protein than cows' milk

3. Regarding the parathyroid gland—
  a. Oxyphil cells secrete parathyroid hormone
  b. Secondary hyperparathyroidism is an inappropriate response to serum calcium levels
  c. Parathyroid hormone is a polypeptide
  d. Low magnesium levels stimulate parathyroid hormone secretion
  e. It secretes calcitonin

4. Concerning iodine—
  a. The minimum daily adult requirement is 500 μg
  b. Is taken up as iodide by the kidneys and thyroid gland
  c. There is an enterohepatic circulation
  d. The iodide pump in the thyroid gland is favoured by an electrical gradient
  e. Thiouracil blocks the binding of iodine to tyrosine

Answers overleaf

1. a. b. d. e.
Insulin is formed as proinsulin in the ribosomes of the rough endoplasmic reticulum of the B cells and stored in the Golgi apparatus. It is initially a single chain polypeptide wih an A-chain at one end and a B-chain at the other end separated by a C peptide. This C peptide is split off to form insulin which is composed of two peptide chains joined by disulphide bonds. Insulin causes decreased lipolysis, increased glycogenosynthesis and increased protein synthesis; its secretion is stimulated by glucagon. In its absence dissolution of fat stores occurs rapidly with diffusion of free fatty acids into the liver. The brain cells are permeable to glucose without the help of insulin.

2. a. c.
Oestrogens are responsible for the development of ducts and progestagens for the development of lobules. Full breast development occurs under the influences of oestrogens, progestagens and prolactin in pregnancy. Oxytocin causes milk ejection by contraction of the myoepithelial cells. Human milk contains 1.2 g/dl of protein whereas cows' milk contains 3.3 g/dl.

3. c. d.
Chief cells secrete parathyroid hormone. The function of oxyphil cells is unclear. Secondary hyperparathyroidism is a wholly appropriate response to low serum calcium levels. Low extracellular concentrations of both magnesium and calcium ions stimulate secretion of parathyroid hormone. Calcitonin is secreted by the parafollicular cells of the thyroid gland.

4. b. c. e.
The minimum daily requirement is 100–150 μg, but the usual intake is 500 μg. Iodide is also taken up by salivary glands, the ciliary body, choroid plexus and breast. Some iodine is excreted in bile and reabsorbed into an enterohepatic circulation. The intracellular space of thyroid cells is 50 mV negative with respect to their extracellular space. The iodide pump works against this gradient.

5. In the thyroid gland—
  a. Thyroglobulin is a polypeptide made of two subunits
  b. Iodide uptake is dependent on Na-K-ATPase activity
  c. Cells secrete a serum calcium-lowering protein
  d. An active gland contains large follicles with abundant colloid
  e. The cells have a prominent endoplasmic reticulum

6. Thyroxine—
  a. Acts via cyclic adenosine monophosphate
  b. Can bind to albumin
  c. Has a half-life of about 7 days
  d. Is mainly metabolized by muscle and liver
  e. Has a biological activity about five times greater than that of tri-iodothyronine

7. Growth hormone—
  a. Is produced by acidophil cells in the anterior pituitary
  b. Shows species-specificity
  c. Acts on growth via somatostatin
  d. Increases plasma glucose concentration
  e. Has a half-life of about 25 minutes

8. Adrenocorticotrophic hormone—
  a. Stimulates aldosterone secretion
  b. Is derived from beta-endorphin
  c. Secretion is increased in Cushing's syndrome caused by adrenal adenoma
  d. Acts by binding to cytoplasmic receptors
  e. Secretion is increased by hypoglycaemia

Answers overleaf

5. b. c. e.
Thyroglobulin is a glycoprotein made of two subunits, its molecular weight being 660 000. Iodine uptake is an active process requiring Na-K-ATPase. Calcitonin is the calcium-lowering hormone secreted by parafollicular C cells of the thyroid. Statement d describes an inactive gland. Active follicles are small and lined by cuboidal or columnar cells. Reabsorption lacunae are a prominent feature. The presence of endoplasmic reticulum is common to most secretory cells.

6. b. c. d.
Thyroxine acts by binding to cytoplasmic receptors which then enter the nucleus to increase expression of messenger RNA. This is followed by translation of the messenger RNA into proteins.

Thyroxine binds to thyroxine-binding globulin and thyroxine-binding prealbumin as well as to albumin in the ratio 60, 30 and 10%. Tri-iodothyronine binds to albumin and thyroxine-binding globulin only.

Tri-iodothyronine has a biological activity five times greater than thyroxine and is probably the active hormone.

7. All
Growth hormone stimulates growth indirectly by causing the liver to produce somatostatin.

Excess of growth hormone in adults produces acromegaly and in children (before fusion of the epiphysis) produces gigantism.

8. e.
Adrenocorticotrophic hormone increases cortisol secretion from the zona fasiculata part of the adrenal cortex. Secretion of aldosterone depends upon the activity of the renin–angiotensin system.

Adrenocorticotrophic hormone is derived from pro-opiomelano-cortin, which gives rise to beta-endorphin. It is a polypeptide of 39 amino acids. It, therefore, acts on surface receptors, which leads to the increase in cyclic adenosine monophosphate.

Adrenocorticotrophic hormone secretion is reduced in adrenal adenoma as a result of negative feedback inhibition on the anterior pituitary gland by cortisol.

9. **Deficiency of the enzyme 21-hydroxylase results in—**
   a. Hypertension
   b. Clitoral hypertrophy
   c. Skin pigmentation
   d. Hyperglycaemia
   e. Hypokalaemic alkalosis

10. **Synthesis of prostaglandins—**
    a. Involves eicosatetraenoic acid
    b. Can be inhibited by indomethacin
    c. Involves a phospholipase
    d. Produces a substance which aggregates platelets
    e. Produces a substance which prevents platelet aggregation

11. **Cortisol—**
    a. Is mainly bound to transcortin in the plasma
    b. Inhibits adrenocorticotrophic hormone
    c. Concentration shows a circadian rhythm with the lowest concentration at 9:00 am
    d. Action leads to glycogen deposition
    e. Is produced by the zona glomerulosa part of the adrenal gland

Answers overleaf

9. b. c.
Deficiency of 21-hydroxylase results in reduced synthesis of cortisol and aldosterone. As a result, the synthetic pathway is diverted to androgen synthesis, which leads to masculinization. The reduced output of cortisol leads to increased secretion of adrenocortico-trophic hormone from the anterior pituitary gland. Adrenocorti-cotrophic hormone is responsible for the increased skin pigmentation.

Deficiency of 17-hydroxylase blocks the synthesis of androgen and diverts the synthetic pathway to cortisol and aldosterone. Therefore, it causes hypertension, hyperglycaemia and hypokalae-mic alkalosis. However, it does not result in masculinization.

10. All
Eicosatetraenoic acid (arachidonic acid) is formed by the action of phospholipase A_2 on membrane phospholipids.

Indomethacin inhibits the cyclo-oxygenase enzyme, not the lipo-oxygenase enzyme. Therefore, synthesis of prostaglandins and thromboxane A_2 is inhibited, but not that of leukotrienes.

Thromboxane A_2 is a very potent aggregator of platelets. Prostacyclin is a very potent antiplatelet aggregating agent. Both substances are derived from arachidonic acid.

11. a. b. d.
Cortisol concentration shows a circadian rhythm with the lowest concentration at midnight.

The zona glomerulosa secretes aldosterone, zona reticularis secretes androgens and zona fasciculata secretes cortisol.

Gastrointestinal

1. **Gastric emptying is inhibited by—**
   a. Gastrin
   b. Hypotonic chyme entering the duodenum
   c. Distension of the duodenal cap
   d. Cholecystokinin
   e. Fear

2. **The following are true of absorption in the gastrointestinal tract—**
   a. Active absorption of calcium occurs mainly in the duodenum
   b. Glucose and galactose compete for the same carrier system
   c. Proteins may be absorbed as di- and tripeptides
   d. Fructose absorption is blocked by metabolic poisons
   e. Bile acids are predominantly absorbed in the terminal ileum

3. **In discussing the function of the gall bladder—**
   a. It is essential for fat digestion
   b. There is a bile salt pool which normally turns over 15–20 times per day
   c. Contraction is enhanced by secretion
   d. It has an acidifying function on bile
   e. It has an innervation from the right posterior branch of the vagus

Answers overleaf

1. b. c. d. e.
Gastric emptying is controlled by the enterogastric reflex. This is under the control of: osmoreceptors and mechanoreceptors in the duodenal cap; the products of protein digestion; and hydrogen ions. Fear, which increases vagal stimulation and cholecystokinin, which is increased due to fat and to a lesser extent protein in the duodenum, inhibits gastric emptying directly. Gastrin expedites gastric emptying as well as increasing the production of acid.

2. a. b. c.
Calcium is poorly absorbed in the intestinal tract because of the relative insolubility of many of its compounds. It is mainly absorbed in the duodenum as an active process. Glucose and galactose are absorbed via the process of cotransport. Whilst most proteins are absorbed as amino acids, di- and tripeptides may be absorbed, which are then converted in the mucosal cells to individual amino acids. Fructose absorption is by facilitated diffusion and so is not affected by metabolic poisons. Bile salts are absorbed in the terminal ileum.

3. d.
The three main functions of the gall bladder are storage, concentration and acidification of bile from the liver. It is not essential for the digestion of fat, as shown by the fact that one can perform a cholecystectomy. There is a normal bile salt pool of about 2–4 g in the normal person which circulates 6–10 times in 24 h as part of the enterophepatic circulation. Absorption of the bile salts occurs by an active process at the internal ileum. This circulation replaces the bile salts that are lost in the faeces every day, which amounts to about 0.6 g over 24 h. The gall bladder may be stimulated to contract via neural and hormonal pathways; the latter, involving cholecystokinin, calcium ions and hydrogen ions, is by far the most important but innervation from the left anterior branch of the vagus may also help.

4. The following are true of bile—
  a. Its electrolyte basis is an alkaline solution resembling that of pancreatic juice
  b. The main primary bile acids are cholic acid and deoxycholic acid
  c. It is concentrated in the gall bladder
  d. Some 50–60% of bile salts are reabsorbed in the terminal ileum
  e. Bile salts entering the colon when the terminal ileum is resected prevent sodium and water reabsorption

5. Secretin–
  a. Causes an increase in pancreatic juice which is rich in enzymes
  b. May augment to the action of cholecystokinin
  c. Secretion is stimulated by the products of protein digestion
  d. Shows marked heterogeneity in its structure
  e. Has no significant effect on the secretion of bile

6. Intestinal smooth muscle—
  a. Has a continuously varying membrane potential
  b. Excitation contraction coupling is fast when compared to heart muscle
  c. Does not require myosin for contraction
  d. Contracts in response to stretch
  e. Responds to acetylcholine via nicotinic receptors

7. During prolonged starvation—
  a. Structural proteins are broken down
  b. The brain utilizes ketone bodies
  c. Glutamate is converted to alpha-ketoglutamate
  d. Fructose 1,6-bisphosphate is converted to fructose 1-phosphate
  e. Acetyl coenzyme A is converted to pyruvate

8. Gastrin release—
  a. Is stimulated by protein in the antral mucosa
  b. Is stimulated by alcohol
  c. Is stimulated by fat in the antral mucosa
  d. Is inhibited if the pH of the antral mucosa falls below 5
  e. Is stimulated by direct action of the vagus nerve

Answers overleaf

4. a. c. e.

The electrolyte basis of bile is similar to that of pancreatic juice, having a pH of between 7.8 and 8.6. This is acidified down to a pH of 7.0–7.4 in the gall bladder where concentration also occurs. The primary bile acids are cholic and chenodeoxycholic acids whereas secondary acids are deoxycholic and lithocholic acids. Some 90–95% of bile salts are reabsorbed in the terminal ileum; if this is prevented, causes osmotic diarrhoea in the colon, which adds to the steatorrhoea caused by the loss of bile salts.

5. b. c.

Secretin is thought to have one structure, in marked contrast to gastrin which has several. It is stimulated by protein digestion and acid. Its main actions are to increase production of alkaline pancreatic juice, to augment the action of cholecystokinin and to decrease acid secretion from the stomach. It may also play a role in pyloric contraction and in increasing insulin secretion. In addition it also helps to increase the secretion of bile.

6. a. d.

Excitation contraction coupling is slow in smooth muscle, the contraction beginning 150 ms after the spike and reaching a peak at 500 ms. In response to stretch, the muscle contracts even in the absence of extrinsic innervation. The cholinergic receptors in smooth muscle are muscarinic.

7. a. b. c. d.

The brain normally uses glucose as the only energy source (like the renal medulla and erythrocytes). However, in prolonged starvation, it can use ketone bodies.

8. a. b. e.

Gastrin release is not stimulated by fat.

The pH of the antral mucosa has to fall below 3 before inhibition of gastrin release occurs.

Pharmacology and general

1. **Iron metabolism—**
   a. Adult males lose about 0.5 g/day
   b. Absorption is inhibited by the ingestion of large amounts of cereals
   c. Ferritin molecules may aggregate in haemosiderosis
   d. In iron deficiency there is a decrease in the levels of transferrin with a simultaneous decrease in its saturation
   e. Idiopathic haemochromatosis is a defect of iron storage

2. **Heparin—**
   a. Is a naturally occurring acidic anticoagulant
   b. Facilitates the action of antithrombin III
   c. May be reversed by the covalent binding of protamine
   d. Is found in the granules of mast cells
   e. Crosses the placenta in pregnancy

3. **Considering diuretics—**
   a. Frusemide acts on both the loop of Henle and diluting segment of the tubule
   b. Diuretics are a common cause of hypokalaemia
   c. Diuretics are a recognized cause of hypouricaemia
   d. Amiloride acts to inhibit aldoserone directly
   e. Urea is an example of an osmotic diuretic

Answers overleaf

1. b. c.
About 0.6 mg of iron is excreted each day by the male, mainly into the faeces. Additional amounts of iron are lost whenever there is bleeding, hence in the female menstrual loss of blood brings an average iron loss of approximately 1.5 mg/day. The average western diet contains 10–15 mg/day, with maximal absorption being 3 mg/day. Iron is predominantly absorbed in the ferrous form in the upper duodenum. It is inhibited by cereal ingestion as these contain large amounts of phytic acid which combines with the iron to form an insoluble compound. After its active absorption iron combines with apoferritin to form ferritin which is the storage form of iron. These molecules may aggregate, especially in lysosomal membranes in haemosiderosis. In iron deficiency there is an increase in the amount of transferrin which is the transport form of iron with a simultaneous decrease in its saturation from its normal value of 33%. Idopathic haemochromatosis is an autosomal recessive disorder where there is a defect of iron absorption.

2. a. b. d. e.
Heparin is a naturally occurring acidic anticoagulant which is found in the granules of mast cells. It facilitates the action of antithrombin III which is a serine protease inhibitor and therefore acts on factors IX, X, XI and XII. Protamine is a highly basic compound which rapidly binds electrochemically with heparin and is used to treat overdosage. Heparin, as opposed to warfarin, crosses the placenta in pregnancy, which is therefore a contraindication to its use.

3. a. b. e.
Frusemide is a very potent diuretic acting on both the loop of Henle and diluting segment of the tubule. It is short-acting and useful both in the non-urgent and urgent situation. A common side-effect of diuretics is hypokalaemia as there is decreased sodium reabsorption in the proximal tubule, thus increasing the sodium load to the distal tubule. This is then reabsorbed at the expense of potassium. Potassium-sparing diuretics such as spironolactone and amiloride act on the distal tubular exchange system. Amiloride acts to inhibit sodium reabsoprtion by interfering with the sodium–potassium pump mechanism. Spironolactone acts by inhibiting aldosterone directly. Some diuretics inhibit renal function to the extent that urate excretion is decreased, thus predisposing to hyperuricaemia and gout.

4. Regarding neuromuscular blockade—
   a. Suxamethonium is a competitive antagonist at the motor endplate
   b. Vecuronium is a depolarizing agent
   c. Neostigmine reverses the effects of non-depolarizing agents
   d. Prolonged apnoea may occur in myasthenia gravis when non-depolarizing agents are used
   e. Suxamethonium is useful for short periods of muscle relaxation

5. Local anaesthetics—
   a. Increase the permeability of membranes to sodium
   b. Tend to affect myelinated fibres before unmyelinated ones
   c. Lignocaine is useful in the treatment of atrial arrhythmias
   d. Will diminish proprioception before pain
   e. May have effects on the central nervous system

6. Agonists of the cholinergic muscarinic receptors include—
   a. Atropine
   b. Muscarine
   c. Pilocarpine
   d. Acetylcholine
   e. Nicotine

7. Agonists at the dopamine receptors include—
   a. Bromocriptine
   b. Apomorphine
   c. Haloperidol
   d. Chlorpromazine
   e. L-dopa

8. Considering folate—
   a. It is destroyed by cooking
   b. The daily requirement is 100 μg
   c. The body reserves may last up to 4 months
   d. The main cause of deficiency in the UK is poor dietary intake
   e. Deficiency may be associated with anticonvulsant therapy

Answers overleaf

4. c. d. e.
Suxamethonium is a depolarizing agent useful for short periods of muscle relaxation. Vecuronium is a non-depolarizing agent and its action is typically reversed by anticholinesterases such as neostigmine. Non-depolarizing agents act as competitive antagonists of aceytlcholine at the endplate.

5. e.
Local anaesthetics decrease membrane permeability to sodium. Autonomic function, touch and pain are lost before proprioception. Central effects include nausea, vomiting, drowsiness and coma. There are also cardiotoxic effects.

6. b. c. d.
Atropine is an antagonist.

Muscarine and pilocarpine are agonists. The latter is used in the treatment of glaucoma as it acts by pupillary constriction.

Acetylcholine acts as agonist on both muscarinic and nicotinic receptors.

Nicotine is an agonist of the nicotinic receptor, not muscarinic receptors.

7. a. b.
Bromocriptine and apomorphine are dopamine receptor agonists. The former is used to treat pituitary microprolactinomas.

Haloperidol and chlorpromazine are dopamine receptor antagonists. They are used as antipsychotic drugs.

L-dopa is a precursor of dopamine.

8. All

9. **Calcium—**
   a. Total plasma levels are about 2.5 mmol/l (10 µg/dl)
   b. Is actively absorbed in the intestine
   c. Given intravenously as a gluconate is useful in the management of hypokalaemia
   d. Some 90% of filtered calcium is reabsorbed in the proximal convoluted tubule
   e. Levels are raised in blood taken from a standing subject

10. **In human pregnancy—**
    a. Fertilization normally takes place in the isthmus of the fallopian tube
    b. Corpus luteum is an important source of progesterone throughout pregnancy
    c. The placenta converts acetate to progesterone
    d. The ovary can convert progesterone to oestrogen directly
    e. The corpus luteum is maintained mainly by ovarian oestrogen

11. **In human parturition—**
    a. Uterine contractility is depressed by oestrogen
    b. Fetal adrenocorticotrophic hormone plays an important role in the control of timing of parturition
    c. Prostaglandin secretion is reduced
    d. Oxytocin is released from the posterior pituitary gland via a spinal reflex, with the afferent information coming from cervical stretch receptors
    e. Prostaglandin can be used to induce abortion

12. **In the secretory phase of the menstrual cycle—**
    a. The plasma oestrogen concentration is at its highest
    b. The plasma progesterone concentration is at its highest
    c. The endometrium contains a large amount of glycogen
    d. Ferning pattern is seen in the cervical mucus
    e. Graafian follicles are found in the ovaries

13. **Concerning male fertility—**
    a. The sperm count is decreased by febrile illness
    b. Sperm motility is decreased in Kartagener's syndrome
    c. Spermatogenesis is inhibited by excess alcohol intake
    d. Azoospermia is usually achieved 2 months after vasectomy
    e. Bilateral ablation of the sympathetic trunks below L2 prevents erection

Answers overleaf

9. a. b. e.
Calcium gluconate may be given to stabilize cardiac cell membranes in hyperkalaemia. Some 60% of filtered calcium is reabsorbed in the proximal tubule, some in the ascending limb of the loop, and the rest in the distal tubule. Distal tubule reabsorption is controlled by parathyroid hormone.

10. d.
Fertilization occurs in the widest part of the fallopian tube – the ampulla. Corpus luteum is maintained by human chorionic gonadotrophin and human chorionic somatomammotrophin. It is only important in early pregnancy to maintain the fertilized ovum by secretion of progesterone. Later in pregnancy, the placenta takes over the function of the corpus luteum.

11. b. d. e.
Uterine contractility is enhanced by oestrogen but depressed by progesterone. Prostaglandin secretion is enhanced and is responsible for uterine contraction.

12. b. c.
The plasma oestrogen concentration is highest in the proliferative phase, where it is responsible for the positive feedback effect on the anterior pituitary gland. This results in the luteinizing hormone surge, which causes ovulation.

The plasma progesterone concentration is highest in the secretory phase. It is responsible for the rise in the basal temperature.

Ferning pattern is seen in the proliferative phase. Graafian follicles are found in the late proliferative phase, prior to ovulation.

13. a. b. c.
Febrile illness in the 2 months prior to testing may lead to low sperm count. In Kartagener's syndrome there is an abnormality in ciliary structure which leads to bronchiectasis, hypomotile sperm and gut malrotation. After vasectomy it takes 3 months or longer to achieve azoospermia. Damage to the sympathetic trunks prevents ejaculation. Erection is governed by the pelvic parasympathetics (nervi erigentes).

14. Considering the testis—
   a. Spermatozoa obtain nourishment from Leydig cells
   b. Low scrotal temperature (34–35°C) decreases the sperm count
   c. There is a blood–testis barrier
   d. Testosterone is secreted by Leydig cells
   e. All spermatozoa contain an X chromosome

15. In thermoregulation—
   a. The sweat glands are innervated by sympathetic cholinergic fibres
   b. Peripheral thermoreceptors are the free nerve endings of A-beta fibres
   c. The core temperature can be measured in the oesophagus, rectum and nasopharynx
   d. Evaporation of 1 g of water is associated with the loss of 0.6 kcal (2.4 kJ) of heat
   e. The rise in the body temperature after ovulation is due to oestrogen

Answers overleaf

14. c. d.
Sertoli cells nourish the spermatozoa. High scrotal temperature (hot baths and tight underwear) lowers the sperm count. There is a blood–testis barrier of unfenestrated capillaries through which proteins penetrate poorly. Sperms are haploid, 50% contain a single Y chromosome and the rest have a single X chromosome.

15. a. c. d.
Periphral thermoreceptors are free nerve endings of A-delta and C fibres. A-beta fibres carry 'touch and pressure' modalities and innervate muscle spindle (flowerspray ending).

The rise in temperature (about 0.5°C) is due to progesterone.

Pathology MCQs

Inflammation and healing

1. **In acute inflammation—**
   a. Pain is partly caused by bradykinin
   b. There is an early migration of macrophages followed by neutrophils
   c. Prostaglandin E_1 may act as a chemotactic agent
   d. Endotoxin activates the alternate pathway of complemenet system
   e. Cyclic guanosine monophosphate enhances chemotaxis

2. **In healing—**
   a. Wound contraction is due to myofibroblasts
   b. Zinc is important
   c. Vitamin C is essential for epidermal proliferation
   d. Keloid results from excessive collagen synthesis
   e. Steroid hormones have a stimulatory effect

3. **Considering the triple response (Lewis)—**
   a. The red reaction is followed by wheal and then by flare
   b. Is the normal response of the tissues to injury
   c. The flare is caused by axonal reflex resulting in dilatation of the adjacent arterioles
   d. The axonal reflex involves antidromic conduction
   e. The wheal is caused by increased permeability to proteins

4. **In a healing fracture—**
   a. There is initially a haematoma followed by an invasion of polymorphs
   b. Woven bone and cartilage may be present simultaneously
   c. The pH of the fracture site is initially acid and later alkaline
   d. Remodelling occurs even after lamellar bone formation
   e. Poor immobilization may result in the formation of an arthrodesis

5. **Wound healing is impaired in the following circumstances—**
   a. Haemolytic anaemia
   b. An arthritic patient on high-dose steroids
   c. Pulsed electromagnetic energy
   d. Environmental temperature of 30°C
   e. The use of modern wound dressings

Answers overleaf

1. a. c. d. e.
There is an early migration of neutrophils followed some hours later by macrophages.

2. a. b. d.
Vitamin C is essential for hydroxylation of proline residues of collagen and the formation of chondroitin sulphate in granulation tissues. Steroid hormones have an inhibitory effect and are used as anti-inflammatory agents and antifibrogenic agents.

3. b. c. d. e.
In Lewis's triple response, the red reaction is caused by increased capillary blood flow due to relaxation of capillary sphincter (mediated by histamine and other chemical mediators). The red reaction occurs within 10 s of the stimulus and.is then followed by the flare response. The wheal response is the last component.

4. a. b. c. d.
The events which follow fracture of a bone are very similar to those of acute inflammation. The haematoma is invade by polymorphs. There then follows a demolition phase, granulation tissue and finally new bone formation. Woven bone laid down by osteoblasts may coexist with cartilage formed by chondroblasts. The changes in pH from acid to alkali may aid bone deposition. Excessive mobility at a fracture site may lead to pseudarthrosis.

5. a. b.
In anaemia there is decreased oxygen delivery to tissues and in haemolysis the raised bilirubin level also impairs healing. Pulsed electromagnetic radiation and ultrasound both promote healing, as does a temperature of 30°C (ideal temperature). Modern dressings allow diffusion of oxygen to the wound, are non-adherent and prevent drying of the wound surface.

6. **The following statements are true of collagen—**
   a. It is formed in granulation tissue by macrophages
   b. A single collagen molecule is composed of helical polypeptide chains
   c. Type II collagen is predominant in cartilage
   d. Vitamin C deficiency results in hydroxylation of proline residues
   e. It is metabolically inert

7. **Cells of the mononuclear phagocytic system include—**
   a. Microglial cells
   b. Kupffer cells
   c. Osteoblasts
   d. Histiocytes
   e. Mast cells

8. **Macrophages—**
   a. Present antigens to T lymphocytes in association with major histocompatibility complex class 1 molecules
   b. May coexist with *Chlamydia*
   c. Are stimulated by lymphokines secreted by B cells
   d. Secrete interleukin-1, an endogenous pyrogen
   e. Secrete interferon

9. **Resolution occurs in the following tissues—**
   a. Liver
   b. Skeletal muscle
   c. Renal tubules
   d. Renal glomeruli
   e. Central nervous system

Answers overleaf

6. b. c.
Collagen is formed by fibroblasts in granulation tissue and is composed of three helical polypeptide chains. Classically, type I collagen is found in bone and tendon, type II in cartilage, type III in cardiovascular structures and types IV and V in basement membranes. However the picture is more complicated than this because types I and III are almost always found together in all tissues apart from cartilage. Vitamin C is required for hydroxylation of proline and lysine residues in collagen. There is a continuous turnover of collagen.

7. a. b. d.
The mononuclear phagocytic system includes cells derived from a bone marrow precursor and capable of avid phagocytosis. Octeoclasts but not osteoblasts are included.

8. b. d. e.
Macrophages present antigens in association with major histocompatibility complex class 2 molecules. Lymphokines (including macrophage chemotactic factor and migration inhibition factor) are secreted by T cells.

9. a. c.
The central nervous system and the skeletal muscles do not regenerate after damage. They are replaced by fibrous tissues.

The liver has a great capacity to regenerate after injury. If persistent injury occurs, then regeneration may be complicated by loss of the normal hepatic architecture, leading to hepatic cirrhosis.

The renal glomeruli do not regenerate, unlike the renal tubules.

10. **Amyloidosis—**
    a. May occur in chronic inflammatory conditions
    b. May cause polyneuropathy
    c. Can be diagnosed by rectal biopsy
    d. Of immune origin is characterized by the presence of an intact heavy chain or its N-terminal
    e. May occur in medullary carcinoma of the thyroid

11. **Granulomas—**
    a. Are formed by collection of neutrophils
    b. Are mediated by cells rather than by serum
    c. May be caused by beryllium
    d. Cannot be caused by helminth infection
    e. Do not contain epithelioid cells

12. **Sarcoidosis—**
    a. Causes parotid gland swelling
    b. Causes condylomata lata
    c. Is associated with the presence of asteroid bodies in the multinucleated giant cells
    d. May cause diabetes insipidus
    e. May cause hypercalcaemia which is not responsive to corticosteroid therapy

13. **The following conditions are recognized causes of aseptic necrosis in bone—**
    a. Decompression sickness
    b. Fracture of the talus
    c. Osteophytes
    d. Fractured neck of femur
    e. Weightlessness

Answers overleaf

10. a. b. c. e.

Amyloid is a fibrillar glycoprotein.

In primary amyloidosis, the heart, gastrointestinal tract, tongue and other muscles are affected.

In secondary amyloidosis, the liver, spleen, kidneys and adrenals are commonly affected. It commonly follows chronic inflammatory conditions such as osteomyelitis, tuberculosis, pyelonephritis, rheumatoid arthritis, leprosy, bronchiectasis and tertiary syphilis. It also follows malignant conditions such as myeloma, Hodgkin's disease, medullary carcinoma of the thyroid gland and leukaemia. Amyloidosis may also be inherited, as in familial Mediterranean fever.

In amyloidosis of immune origin, the amyloid protein consists of the light chain part of immunoglobulins.

11. b. c.

Granulomas are nodular aggregates of mature monocytes and epithelioid macrophages. They may be caused by beryllium or helminth infection.

12. a. c. d.

Condylomata lata are flat papules found in the cutaneous and mucocutaneous areas of perineum in cases of secondary syphilis.

Sarcoid-induced hypercalcaemia is responsive to corticosteroid treatment. It is hyperparathyroidism-induced hypercalcaemia which is not responsive to corticosteroid therapy.

13. a. b. d.

Aseptic (avascular) necrosis occurs in 'the bends' (decompression sickness), sickle cell disease and in certain fractures which destroy the blood supply to a bone, e.g. scaphoid, talus, neck of femur. Though weightlessness causes osteoporosis which makes bone less resistant to fracture, weightlessness *per se* does not cause aseptic necrosis.

Neoplasia

1. The following are tumours of bone—
a. Osteosarcoma
b. Ameloblastoma
c. Ewing's tumour
d. Malignant fibrous histocytoma
e. Chordoma

2. Carcinoma of the cervix—
a. Occurs predominantly at the squamocolumnar junction on the ectocervix
b. Is mainly of the adenocarcinoma type
c. May occur as carcinoma-*in-situ*
d. Occurs more commonly in nulliparous women
e. Metastasizes early to the liver

3. In benign prostatic hyperplasia—
a. Histologically there is adenosis and epitheliosis
b. There is no association with bladder diverticula
c. There may be an unexpected malignancy in approximately 10% of surgically removed prostates
d. Haematuria may be a presenting symptom
e. Renal failure is a recognized complication

Answers overleaf

1. All
Osteosarcoma is a tumour of osteoblasts of bimodal age distribution, commonest in the age group 10–25. In an old age group it may arise in association with Paget's disease. Ameloblastoma is a locally invasive tumour derived from the epithelial cells of the enamel organ. It usually involves the lower jaw towards its angle where gradual destruction in the jaw takes place but the tumour metastasizes only rarely. Ewing's tumour is a progessive childhood tumour of unknown origin. Chordoma is a rare tumour resulting from the remnants of the notochord usually found in the sacrococcygeal area or base of the skull.

2. a. c.
Carcinoma of the cervix is predominantly squamous in type and arises mainly from the squamocolumnar junction which as the cervix grows moves out from the endocervix to the ectocervix. Only 5% of tumours are adenocarcinoma in type. The main aetiological factors revolve around early sexual intercourse, promiscuity and low social class, hence multiparous women more commonly have cervical carcinoma. Carcinoma of the cervix usually spreads directly and then to local lymph nodes; only rarely does it metastasize to the liver.

3. a. b. d. e.
Benign prostatic hyperplasia is common over the age of 50 and consists of an increased number of glands (adenosis) and an increase in the number of cells forming these new glands (epitheliosis). Prostatic obstruction increases the resistance in the flow of urine, so causing detrusor muscle hypertrophy. Between hypertrophied fibres saccules and diverticula may form. Later back-pressure of urine up the ureters may cause postrenal failure. A drop of blood at the beginning or end of micturition is not unusual. Marked haematuria may result from rupture of an engorged prostatic venous plexus.

4. Malignant melanomas—
   a. Do not occur on the palms or soles
   b. Have a better prognosis in women
   c. Do not metastasize to the skin
   d. Have a worse prognosis in pregnancy
   e. In males are commonest on the trunk

5. Concerning carcinoma of the breast—
   a. It is most commonly found in the upper outer quadrant of the breast
   b. In the TNM system T1 describes a tumour up to 3 cm in diameter
   c. About 30% of carcinomas are hormone-dependent
   d. An accurate prognostic factor is the histological status of axillary nodes
   e. Cancer of the male breast accounts for 5% of breast carcinoma

6. Malignant tumours have the following characteristics
   a. Invasiveness
   b. Anaplasia
   c. High nuclear to cytoplasmic ratio
   d. Fibrous reaction of the stroma
   e. Abnormal mitoses

7. Pituitary tumours—
   a. Include chromophobe adenoma, which commonly secretes adrenocorticotrophic hormone
   b. Include eosinophil adenoma, which commonly secretes growth hormone to produce gigantism in children and acromegaly in adults
   c. Include basophil adenoma, which commonly secretes prolactin
   d. Include craniopharyngioma, which is derived from Rathke's pouch
   e. May present with diabetes insipidus

Answers overleaf

4. b. e.
Malignant melanomas may occur anywhere in the body, commonly on the lower leg in the female and trunk in the male. Peripheral lesions in general have a better prognosis, although the disease does not appear to be influenced by hormone therapy. Pregnancy may make pigmented moles darker and sometimes larger but does not affect the course of malignant melanomas. Blood-borne metastases may be seen in the lungs, liver, brain, bones and skin and less commonly at the small intestine and heart.

5. a. c. d.
About 60% of carcinomas are found in the upper outer quadrant. In the TNM system T1 tumours are less than 2 cm in diameter. Hormone-dependent tumours are responsive to therapy by alteration of the hormonal milieu, e.g. with tamoxifen. These tumours account for about 30% of breast carcinomas. The histological state of axillary lymph nodes as determined by surgical sampling is said to be a very accurate measure of the prognosis. Cancer of the male breast accounts for less than 2% of breast cancers.

6. a. b. c. e.
Fibrous reaction is rare in malignant tumours (e.g. scirrhous carcinoma of the breast).

Anaplasia is a characteristic feature as the tumours do not resemble their parent tissues.

Abnormal mitoses and increased mitoses occur, which result in an increased nuclear to cytoplasmic ratio.

7. b. d. e.
Chromophobe adenoma is commonly non-secreting and exerts its effect by compressing the optic chiasm and other parts of the pituitary gland. Basophil adenoma commonly secretes adrenocorticotrophic hormone, which causes Cushing's syndrome.

8. Phaeochromocytoma—
 a. Is malignant in 90% of cases
 b. Can produce sustained hypertension
 c. Is associated with pancreatic tumour
 d. Is associated with medullary carcinoma of the thyroid gland
 e. Is found in the adrenal gland in 90% of cases

9. Carcinoid tumours—
 a. Are found most commonly in the terminal ileum
 b. Are found in the lung
 c. Produce the carcinoid syndrome only when metastases occur in the liver
 d. Are made up of Kulchitsky cells, which take up silver stains
 e. Are diagnosed by estimation of urinary 5-hydroxyindole acetic acid

10. Predisposing factors of carcinoma of the oesophagus include—
 a. Pharyngeal pouch
 b. Achalasia of the cardia
 c. Caustic stricture
 d. Plummer–Vinson syndrome
 e. Reflux oesophagitis

11. The following pairings of tumours and their causes are correct—
 a. 2-Naphthylamine and bladder carcinoma
 b. Benzene and leukaemia
 c. Hardwood dusts and adenocarcinoma of the paranasal sinuses
 d. Aflatoxin and liver cell carcinoma
 e. Cyclophosphamide and leukaemia

12. The following conditions are associated with malignant tumours—
 a. Acanthosis nigricans
 b. Erythmea nodosum
 c. Dermatomyositis
 d. Erythema gyratum repens
 e. Eaton–Lambert syndrome

Answers overleaf

8. b. d. e.
Phaeochromocytoma can be regarded as the '10% tumour'. It is malignant in 10% of cases; is bilateral in 10% of cases; and is found outside the adrenal gland in 10% of cases.

It can produce sustained or intermittent hypertension.

Phaeochromocytoma is associated with medullary carcinoma of the thyroid gland and nodular parathyroid adenoma, as part of the multiple endocrine neoplastic syndrome type 2. Phaeochromocytoma is also associated with neurofibromata, as part of the von Recklinghausen syndrome.

9. b. c. d. e.
The most common site of carcinoid tumours is the appendix, but it can be found anywhere in the gastrointestinal tract and the lung.

10. b. c. d.
Reflux oesophagitis may be complicated by Barrett's oesophagitis.

Plummer–Vinson syndrome is the association between an oesophageal web causing dysphagia and iron-deficiency anaemia. It predisposes to postcricoid carcinoma.

Other predisposing factors of oesphageal carcinoma include tylosis and smoking.

11. All

12. a. c. d. e.
Erythema nodosum consists of painful, nodular erythematous lesions on the shins. It is commonly associated with infections (streptococcus, mycobacterium and leprosy), sarcoid, and drugs (sulphonamide, dapsone and oral contraceptives). Acanthosis nigricans consists of pigmented thickening of the skin of the axilla or groin with warty lesions. It is commonly associated with carcinoma of the stomach.

Eaton–Lambert syndrome consists of myasthenia like symptoms in association with bronchial carcinoma.

13. **The following conditions predispose to squamous cell carcinoma—**
    a. Bowen's disease
    b. Senile keratosis
    c. Keratoacanthoma
    d. Lupus vulgaris
    e. Chronic ulceration

Answers overleaf

13. a. b. d. e.
Keratoacanthoma is a benign skin condition and does not predispose to squamous cell carcinoma.

Microbiology

1. **The following viruses can produce malignant tumours in humans—**
   a. Human papillomavirus
   b. Herpes simplex virus type 2
   c. Hepatitis A virus
   d. Hepatitis B virus
   e. Epstein–Barr virus

2. **Concerning antibiotics—**
   a. The cephalosporins act to prevent bacterial cell wall synthesis
   b. Amphotericin is an antifungal drug acting on the cell membrane
   c. Chloramphenicol is a wide-spectrum bacteriostatic antibiotic
   d. Ciprofloxacin affects RNA production and is effective agains *Pseudomonas aeruginosa*
   e. The cerebrospinal fluid is easily accessible to penicillins

3. **In hydatid disease—**
   a. It is usually caused by the larval stage of the *Echinococcus tapeworm*
   b. Humans are infected by larvae penetrating their skin
   c. The adult worm lives harmlessly in the dog intestine
   d. Cysts may occur in the brain and bone
   e. There is a danger of anaphylaxis if a hepatic cyst ruptures

4. **Amoebic liver abscess—**
   a. Is caused by *Entamoeba coli*
   b. Is best treated by metronidazole
   c. Is best treated by continuous percutaneous drainage
   d. Is best treated by tetracycline
   e. Is sterile

5. *Staphylococcus aureus*—
   a. Is an aerobic and facultatively anaerobic Gram-positive coccus found in clusters
   b. Is a catalase-negative organism
   c. Coagulates fibrinogen
   d. May cause food poisoning following the ingestion of an endotoxin
   e. May be found on the umbilicus of the newborn

Answers overleaf

1. a. b. d. e.
Human papillomavirus and herpes simplex virus type 2 are
implicated in the pathogenesis of cervical carcinoma.
  Hepatitis B virus is involved in the pathogenesis of hepatic
carcinoma. Hepatitis A virus is not implicated.
  Epstein–Barr virus causes infectious mononucleosis in western
countries. However, in the malaria-endemic regions of Africa, it is
responsible for the high incidence of Burkitt's lymphoma.

2. a. b. c.
Ciprofloxacin is a quinoline which acts to prevent DNA synthesis,
Rifampicin acts on RNA production. Penicillin does not easily
penetrate the cerebrospinal fluid and so needs to be administered in
high doses.

3. a. c. d. e.
Hydatid disease is caused by the dog tapeworm *Echinococcus
granularis*. The ova are ingested after direct or indirect contact with
dog faeces and are carried in the blood to the liver, lungs, spleen,
bones and brain. Hydatid cysts may be single or multiple and may
cause anaphylaxis if they rupture.

4. b. e.
Amoebic liver abscess is caused by *Entamoeba histolytica*. Amoebic
liver abscess is often sterile on bacteriological culture.

5. c. e.
Staphylococcus aureus is an aerobic and facultatively anaerobic
Gram-positive coccus found in grape-like bunches. They are
catalase-positive, so distinguishing them from the catalase–
negative streptococcus. They are also coagulase-positive, hence
coagulating fibrinogen, this feature distinguishing them from
Staphylococcus epidermidis which is coagulase negative. Food
poisoning is due to the release of an exotoxin which is a protein
which exerts specific effects on selective tissue. This organism may
be found on the umbilicus of the newborn but is most commonly
found in the anterior nares of healthy people.

6. Concerning fungal infections—
  a. Fungi are prokaryotic organisms
  b. *Trichophyton rubrum* is a common cause of tinea pedis
  c. Griseofulvin is an oral fungistatic drug which penetrates mature keratin
  d. Systemic candidal infection may lead to characteristic soft white retinal plaques
  e. Infection with *Cryptococcus neoforms* may cause chronic meningoencephalitis

7. The following species are Gram-positive—
  a. *Bacteroides*
  b. *Actinomyces*
  c. *Listeria*
  d. *Pseudomonas*
  e. *Branhamella*

8. These statements are true of *Clostridium tetani* infection—
  a. The organism is a Gram-positive anaerobe with a central spore
  b. The endotoxin travels along motor nerves to the anterior horn cells
  c. Tetanus may occur weeks to months after the initial inefection
  d. An X-ray shows gas in the subcutaneous tissues and muscles
  e. Tetanus antitoxin is effective once the toxin becomes fixed in nervous tissue

Answers overleaf

6. b. d. e.

Fungi constitute a large ubiquitous group of heterotrophic eukaryotic (DNA organized in nuclei) microorganisms. Tinea pedis is one of the forms of dermatophytosis, which are commonly caused by the *Trychophyton, Microsporum* and *Epidermophyton* species which invade the stratum corneum of the skin, nails and hair shafts. Systemic candidal infections are a serious infection most often seen in the debilitated and immunocompromized. There may be foci in the retina, then in the meninges, brain, kidney, muscle and heart valves. *Cryptococcus neoformans,* usually found in the droppings of pigeons, mainly causes disease of the lungs but may be spread via the blood stream to the meninges. Griseofulvin is an important oral antifungal drug which is concentrated in the outer stratum corneum. It does not penetrate mature keratin or affect a fungus established in it. For this reasons treatment must be continued until all the infected tissue has grown out.

7. b. c.

The Gram stain is a simple, easy-to-perform test which is very important for distinguishing between different bacterias. In the test methyl violet is poured on to a bacterial smear which is fixed by gentle heat and then secured by a solution of iodine. This is then washed with alcohol, acetone, and counter-stained. Gram-negative organisms are decolorized and are not easily visible, while the Gram-positive bacteria retain the original violet stain. *Pseudomonas* is an aerobic rod whereas *Branhamella* is an aerobic coccus; *Bacteroides* is an anaerobic road – all three are Gram-negative. *Listeria* is an aerobic, non-sporing rod whereas *Actinomyces* is an anaerobic branching organism.

8. c.

Clostridium tetani is a Gram-positive anaerobe with a terminal spore (drumstick appearance). It infects wounds contaminated with soil and faeces. In the presence of dead tissue in anaerobic conditions the spores germinate and produce a powerful exotoxin. The toxin travels along motor nerves and, once fixed in nervous tissue, is safe from neutralization by the antitoxin. Gas in the tissues is a feature of infection by *Clostridium perfringens, C. oedematiens* and *C. speticum.*

9. **The following causes of food poisoning result from exotoxins—**
   a. *Shigella* dysentery
   b. *Staphylococcus aureus*
   c. Cholera
   d. *Clostridium perfringens*
   e. Typhoid fever

10. **Pathogenic factors of bacteria include—**
    a. Protein A of *Staphylococcus aureus*
    b. IgA$_1$ protease of *Streptococcus pyogenes*
    c. Epidermolytic toxin of *Staphylococcus aureus*
    d. Coagulase of *Streptococcus pyogenes*
    e. Polysaccharide capsule of *Streptococcus pneumoniae*

11. **Actinomycosis—**
    a. Involves infection by anaerobic filamentous bacteria
    b. May result in chronic purulent infection in humans
    c. Most commonly affects the perineum
    d. May be associated with the presence of an intrauterine contraceptive device
    e. May affect the vermiform appendix

12. **Considering viral hepatitis—**
    a. It may be caused by the Epstein–Barr virus
    b. HBsAg is infective
    c. Persistence of anti-HBs (antibody to HBsAg) indicates a high risk of developing chronic liver disease
    d. The agent of hepatitis B is a DNA virus
    e. It may result in centrilobular necrosis

13. **The following vaccines are live vaccines—**
    a. Diphtheria vaccine
    b. Rabies vaccine
    c. BCG
    d. Tetanus vaccine
    e. Typhoid vaccine

14. **DNA-containing viruses include—**
    a. Poxoviruses
    b. Paramyxoviruses
    c. Rhabdoviruses
    d. Herpesviruses
    e. Papovaviruses

Answers overleaf

9. b. c. d.
Shigella is invasive and does not produce an exotoxin.
Typhoid fever is caused by *Salmonella typhi* or *S. paratyphi*.

10. a. c. e.
IgA$_1$ protease is found in *Neisseria gonorrhoeae* or *N. menigitidis* but not in *Streptococcus pyogenes*.
Coagulase is found in *Staphylococcus aureus*, not in *Streptococcus pyogenes*.

11. a. b. d. e.
This filamentous anaerobic bacterium causes chronic purulent infection in humans and may be the cause of pelvic inflammatory disease when associated with an intrauterine device. Actinomycosis commonly affects the jaw and buccal area.

12. a. d. e.
The agent of hepatitis B is a DNA virus. The HbsAg is not itself infective. The persistence of HBsAg indicates a risk of developing chronic liver disease. Viral hepatitis usually causes centrilobular (zone 3) necrosis.

13. c.
Tetanus and diphtheria vaccines are toxoids.
Rabies and typhoid vaccines are 'killed' vaccines.
Please note that there is a new attenuated *Salmonella typhi* vaccine becoming available.

14. a. d. e.
Paramyxoviruses are RNA-containing viruses which cause sore throats and croup (parainfluenza virus), mumps, measles and lower respiratory tract infection (respiratory syncytial virus).
Rhabdoviruses contain single-stranded RNA. They include the rabies virus.

15. Interferon—
   a. Release is triggered by endotoxin
   b. Induced by virus infection is species-specific
   c. Induced by virus infection is virus-specific
   d. Production is stimulated by viral protein
   e. Produces its effect by blocking the translation of viral messenger RNA in the host cell polyribosomes

16. Treponema pallidum—
   a. Causes condylomata lata
   b. Causes painful chancre as the primary lesion
   c. Can be found in lesions of patients with primary syphilis
   d. Can be found in lesions of patients with secondary syphilis
   e. Causes general paralysis of the insane

17. Congenital syphilis—
   a. Causes deformities of bones
   b. Causes interstitial fibrosis of the lung
   c. Causes deformity of the teeth
   d. Causes fibrosis of the liver
   e. Causes inflammation of the cornea

18. The Wasserman complement fixation test may be positive in—
   a. Yaws
   b. Malaria
   c. Pregnancy
   d. *Mycoplasma* pneumonia
   e. Autoimmune haemolytic anaemia

Answers overleaf

15. a. b. e.
Interferon induced by virus infection is not virus-specific but is species-specific.

Production of interferon is stimulated by foreign double-stranded RNA not viral protein.

16. a. c. d. e.
Chancre is a painless primary lesion of *Treponema pallidum*.

The organism can be found in primary and in secondary syphilitic lesions but not in the blood or cerebrospinal fluid of patients with tertiary syphilis.

17. All
Congenital syphilis causes all of the above problems.

18. All
The Wasserman test is positive in treponemal diseases such as yaws, pinta, bejel and syphilis. False positives occur in conditions b–e, infectious mononucleosis and systemic lupus erythematosus.

Haematology

1. Concerning thrombocytopenia—
a. Spontaneous bleeding rarely occurs unless the platelet count is less than 20 × 109/1
b. It may be helped by administration of vitamin K
c. If of idiopathic type, it usually runs a chronic course in both adults and children
d. It may be associated with diuretic therapy
e. It may occur in von Willebrand's disease

2. Primary polycythaemia—
a. Is an example of a myeloproliferative disorder
b. May present with splenomegaly and pruritis
c. Has a well-recognized tendency to transform to myelofibrosis
d. Is not usually treated with busulphan
e. May have an associated thrombocytosis

3. Chronic lymphatic leukaemia—
a. Has a predominantly bimodal age distribution affecting the young and middle-aged
b. Is the commonest form of leukaemia
c. Is characterized by an absolute lymphocytosis of 10–20 × 10^9 WBC/l
d. May transform to an acute leukaemia
e. Most cases are T-cell in origin

4. Macrocytosis in the peripheral blood film is caused by—
a. Iron deficiency
b. Folate deficiency
c. Alcoholism
d. Vitamin B_{12} deficiency
e. Beta-thalassaemia

Answers overleaf

1. a. c. d.
Thrombocytopenia is a disease of decreased platelet numbers in which spontaneous bleeding rarely occurs unless the platelet count is below 20 or often below 10 × 10^9/l. The cause can usually be attributed to either a failure of production (aplastic anaemia, myelodysplasia, myelofibrosis, malignant infiltrations) or an increased destruction, i.e. autoimmune, drug-induced and hypersplenism. In idiopathic thrombocytopenia the disease usually runs a self-limiting course in children. Diuretics and other drugs such as quinine and sulphonamides often act as a hapten: the drug–antibody complex is passively absorbed on to platelets. In von Willebrand's disease there is an abnormality of platelet function.

2. a. b. c. e.
The myeloproliferative disorders are disorders of totipotential or committed myeloid stem cells, including the eyrthroblasts, megakaryocytes and fibroblasts. Overlap and transformations may occur with 30% chance of transformation to myelofibrosis and a 15% chance of transformation to acute myeloid leukaemia. One of the mainstays of treatment is busulphan and the disease may have an associated high neutrophil and/or platelet count.

3. b.
Chronic lymphatic leukaemia is a lymphoproliferative disorder mainly affecting the elderly, although it may occur in a younger age group. It is characterized by an absolute lymphocytosis of 20–200 × 10^9 WBC/l with or without lymphadenopathy and/or splenomegaly. It is usually B-cell in origin but transformation to acute leukaemia does not occur, although it may transform to an aggressive lymphoma.

4. b. c. d.
Iron deficiency and beta-thalassaemia cause microcytosis in the peripheral blood film.
   Other causes of macrocytosis in the peripheral blood film include: hypothyroidism, pregnancy, chronic respiratory failure and leukoerythroblastic anaemia.

5. Agranulocytosis—
   a. The white cell count is below $2 \times 10^9/l$ (2000/μl)
   b. Is caused by carbimazole
   c. Leads to recurrent viral infections
   d. Is associated with necrotic lesions of the skin
   e. Predisposes to calf vein thrombosis

6. Concerning the spleen—
   a. Splenectomy leads to an immediate neutrophil leukocytosis
   b. It is important in defending against *Haemophilus septicaemia*
   c. Hypersplenism is a cause of leukocytosis
   d. It is enlarged in schistosomiasis
   e. Splenectomy is indicated in hereditary spherocytosis

Answers overleaf

5.   a. b. d.
Carbimazole and sulphonamides are important causes of agranu-locytosis. The condition leads to recurrent bacterial infections because of the low numbers of phagocytic cells present. Necrotic skin lesions contain lymphocytes and plasma cells but few, if any, polymorphs. There is no link with deep venous thrombosis.

6.   a. b. d. e.
The immediate neutrophil leukocytosis following splenectomy is greater than can be attributed merely to a surgical procedure. The spleen contains cells which are able to phagocytose organisms in the absence of opsonizing antibodies, and the organ is important in mounting a defence against blood-borne infections, the pneumo-coccus being the best example. Hypersplenism is a cause of pancytopenia rather than leukocytosis. Hereditary spherocytosis is the indication *par excellence* for splenectomy in the absence of trauma.

General

1. **Hyperuricaemia occurs in—**
   a. Psoriasis
   b. Probenecid
   c. Toxaemia of pregnancy
   d. Thiazide diuretics
   e. Diabetic ketoacidosis

2. **Isoenzymes of alkaline phosphatase are found in—**
   a. Erythrocytes
   b. Liver
   c. Bone
   d. Gut
   e. Placenta

3. **Considering jaundice—**
   a. It is usually apparent clinically when serum bilirubin is 20 μmol/l
   b. Unconjugated bilirubin is water-soluble
   c. Urine is usually bile-stained in Gilbert's syndrome
   d. It may be encountered in pregnancy
   e. Bile ductular proliferation in portal tracts is a feature of obstruction of large bile ducts

4. **Hypercalcaemia occurs in—**
   a. Thyrotoxicosis
   b. Sarcoidosis
   c. Secondary hyperparathyroidism
   d. Immobilized Paget's disease
   e. Addison's disease

5. **Atherosclerosis—**
   a. Cannot be produced in experimental animals
   b. May lead to a sudden arterial obstruction
   c. Is the main cause of false aneurysms
   d. Is commonly associated with polyarteritis nodosa
   e. Occurs in pulmonary arteries

Answers overleaf

1. a. c. d. e.
Urate is the endproduct of the breakdown of purines from nucleic acids. Increased levels may be caused by increased rate of urate formation or by reduced rate of excretion. Urate filters through the glomerulus, after which most is reabsorbed in the tubular lumen. Over 80% is then actively secreted back into the lumen. The acetoacetate molecules which may result from diabetic ketoacidosis compete for this active mechanism. Thiazide diuretics themselves also inhibit urate excretion. Probenecid is used in the treatment of hyperuricaemia as it increases secretion.

2. b. c. d. e.
Alkaline phosphatase is commonly found in disorders of liver and bone. It is also increased in pregnancy. Aspartate transaminase and lactate dehydrogenase are found in erythrocytes.

3. d. e.
Jaundice becomes clinically apparent at about 35 μmol/l of bilirubin. Gilbert's syndrome is due to a defect in the uptake of unconjugated bilirubin. This is not water-soluble so does not appear in the urine. The jaundice of pregnancy occurs typically in the last trimester and may be caused by the high level of oestrogens.

4. a. b. d. e.
Secondary hyperparathyroidism is the response of the parathyroid glands to hypocalcaemia. The raised parathyroid hormone is therefore appropriate to the low plasma calcium concentration. This occurs commonly in chronic renal failure or vitamin D deficiency.

5. b. e.
Atherosclerosis has been produced in several animals including the rabbit and pigeon. Gradual arterial obstruction is the usual sequel to atheroma but haemorrhage into a plaque or thrombosis on an ulcerated plaque may cause sudden obstruction. In pulmonary hypertension atherosclerotic plaques may be found in the pulmonary arteries.

6. **Deep venous thrombosis—**
   a. Is a specific postoperative complication of splenectomy
   b. Begins with the formation of coralline thrombus
   c. Forms during the course of a long operation
   d. Is a recognized feature of hyperthyroidism
   e. Is diagnosed effectively by clinical examination

7. **Gaseous embolism may occur in the following circumstances—**
   a. Operations on the neck
   b. The insertion of orthopaedic cement
   c. Travel in unpressurized aircraft
   d. Rapid descent in a deep sea dive
   e. The intravenous infusion of fluids

8. **The following are causes of osteoporosis—**
   a. Prolonged heparin therapy
   b. Thyrotoxicosis
   c. Diabetes mellitus
   d. Alcoholism
   e. Cytotoxic drugs

9. **Woven bone is normally found in—**
   a. The developing clavicle of fetus
   b. The adult clavicle
   c. Cancellous bone of the proximal femur
   d. The granulation tissue of a healing fracture
   e. Osteogenic tumours

10. **The following are recognized causes of cirrhosis of the liver—**
    a. Haemochromatosis
    b. Galactosaemia
    c. *Clonorchis sinensis* infection
    d. Carbon tetrachloride poisoning
    e. Methotrexate

Answers overleaf

6. a. c.
Deep venous thrombosis is a common postoperative complication, especially in splenectomy because of the rise in the number of platelets. It often begins during the course of a long operation with the formation of platelet thrombus followed by coralline thrombus. Clinical diagnosis is probably no more than 50% accurate in deep venous thrombosis.

7. a. b. e.
If the patient is in the head-up position such that the veins of the neck are collapsed, an incision into the veins will allow air at atmospheric pressure to be sucked into circulation. Pushing cement into the medullary cavity of bone may force trapped air into the medullary vessels and thence into the circulation. Air embolism occurs rarely with modern intravenous giving sets but is still a possibility. Rapid ascent, but not descent, from a dive, may cause embolism.

8. All
Common causes of osteoporosis include steroid therapy, the postmenopausal state and immobility.

9. a. d. e.
Woven bone is usually found in sites where membranous ossification is taking place, in healing fractures and in osteogenic tumours. The adult clavicle and proximal femur consist of lamellar bone.

10. a. b. e.
Cirrhosis describes the process of diffuse hepatic fibrosis with regeneration nodules and may be caused by methotrexate and the familiar disorder of galactose metabolism. Haemochromatosis may cause cirrhosis as there is an increased deposition of iron in the liver parenchyma. Carbon tetrachloride is associated with centrilobular hepatic necrosis and the liver fluke *Clonorchis sinensis* is associated with cholangiocarcinoma.

11. **Hepatic fatty change may occur in—**
    a. Diabetes mellitus
    b. Obesity
    c. Kwashiorkor
    d. Ulcerative colitis
    e. Alcohol abuse

12. **In nephrocalcinosis—**
    a. There is typically diffuse calcification in the renal cortex
    b. The patient may have medullary sponge kidney
    c. There may be renal tubular acidosis
    d. Hyperthyroidism is a cause
    e. There is dystrophic calcification of the kidneys

13. **Concerning renal calculi—**
    a. They may be a complication of hyperparathyroidism
    b. They may be a complication of chemotherapy
    c. Oxalate stones are usually due to a metabolic disorder
    d. Xanthine stones characteristically have a sharp surface
    e. They are increasingly found in the acidic urine associated with *Proteus* infections

14. **Metastatic calcification occurs in—**
    a. Tuberculosis
    b. Fat necrosis
    c. Atherosclerotic plaque
    d. Primary hyperthyroidism
    e. Renal tubular acidosis

Answers overleaf

11. All
Hepatic fatty change or steatosis is the deposition of fat droplets in the cytoplasm due to many insults. It is usually reversible and does not by itself result in progression to other conditions such as cirrhosis.

12. b. c. d.
Diffuse calcification in the renal cortex is present in less than 5% of cases so it is not a typical feature. Hyperthyroidism and renal tubular acidosis account for 60% of cases. Medullary sponge kidney is another important cause of nephrocalcinosis. Dystrophic calcification occurs in abnormal tissue in the presence of normal serum calcium levels. In most of the cases of nephrocalcinosis the serum calcium is elevated and there is metastatic calcification.

13. a. b.
Calculi may complicate the hypercalciuria of predominantly primary or tertiary hyperparathyroidism. Oxalate stones are often referred to as idiopathic stones and are not usually due to a metabolic disorder. They may be caused by an imbalance in the calcium oxalate concentration as well as altered urinary pH. *Proteus* splits urea so releasing ammonia and tends to cause the urine to become alkaline. Chemotherapy causes increased cell breakdown, with the release of many constituents into the blood, and may be responsible for renal calculi, e.g. urate stones. Xanthine stones are rare and tend to be smooth and round as opposed to oxalate stones which are characteristically sharp and mulberry-shaped.

14. d. e.
Metastatic calcification is associated with high blood calcium levels and therefore does not occur in tuberculosis, fat necrosis or atherosclerotic plaque.

15. **The following are true of acute pancreatitis—**
    a. There is an association with cholelithiasis
    b. It may complicate infection with certain paramyxoviruses
    c. A serum amylase level is not a specific test in diagnosis
    d. There may be glycosuria in over 30% of cases
    e. There may be clinically occult respiratory failure in the first few days

16. **Regarding the stomach—**
    a. Gastric erosions penetrate the muscularis mucosae
    b. Cushing's ulcers occur typically in burns patients
    c. Necrosis of the lesser curve may occur after gastric vagotomy
    d. In infantile pyloric stenosis there is both hyperplasia and hypertrophy
    e. Gastric carcinoma has a greater incidence in people of blood group O

17. **Tumour necrosis factor—**
    a. Is a protein produced by neoplastic cells
    b. Is produced in response to endotoxin
    c. Prevents the production of hydrogen peroxide by neutrophils
    d. Is a cytokine
    e. Antibodies may prolong allograft survival

18. **Melanin—**
    a. Is synthesized from tyrosine
    b. Is found in substantia nigra
    c. Production is stimulated by adrenocorticotrophic hormone
    d. Is responsible for the focal pigmentation of the lips in Peutz-Jeghers syndrome
    e. Is responsible for the pigmentation found in neurofibromatosis

19. **The following are recognized associations—**
    a. Berry aneurysms and infantile polycystic renal disease
    b. Cirrhosis of the liver and haemochromatosis
    c. Subacute bacterial endocarditis and *Streptococcus viridans*
    d. Interstitial pulmonary fibrosis and bleomycin
    e. Squamous cell carcinoma of the skin and senile keratosis

Answers overleaf

15. a. b. c. e.
Gall stones are commonly associated with acute pancreatitis, as is excessive alcohol consumption. The mumps paramyxovirus usually causes interstitial tissue inflammation. Amylase levels are not specific and may be increased in perforated peptic ulcer, coronary thrombosis, intestinal obstruction, and may also be raised if morphia or codeine has been given to the patient. Glycosuria tends to occur in only 10–15% of patients. Acute pancreatitis may lead to multisystem failure, respiratory failure may be overt and it is therefore important to do arterial blood gases on admission.

16. c. d. e.
Gastric erosions are superficial to the muscularis mucosae. Curling's ulcers occur in burns patients and Cushing's in head injuries. Blood group O and peptic ulcer are associated, but gastric carcinoma is associated with group A. Necrosis of the lesser curve after vagotomy is probably secondary to devascularization of the lesser curve.

17. b. d. e.
Tumour necrosis factor is a cytokine produced by activated macrophages, lymphocytes and vascular smooth muscle. The lipopolysaccharide of endotoxin is the most potent stimulus of endotoxin production. Tumour necrosis factor stimulates hydrogen peroxide production by neutrophils and prevents the clonal expansion of cells responsible for graft rejection.

18. All

19. b. c. d. e.
Berry aneurysms are the commonest cause of subarachnoid haemorrhage and are thought to be congenital in nature. They can be solitary or multiple or even symmetrical and have known associations with coarctation of the aorta, adult-type polycystic renal disease and renal artery stenosis. Cirrhosis of the liver is a sequel of haemochromatosis where there is increased iron absorption.

20. Consider the following statements. True or false?—

    a.   Repair is a process whereby lost tissue is replaced by tissue of the same type

    b.   Atrophy is a decrease in the size or number of cells in a tissue

    c.   Hypoplasia is a recognized precursor of neoplasia

    d.   Squamous metaplasia occurs only in squamous epithelium

    e.   In hyperplasia there is an abnormal nuclear to cytoplasmic ratio

Answers overleaf

20. b.
The first statement describes regeneration. Strictly speaking, repair is replacement by scar tissue. Squamous metaplasia may occur in epithelia other than squamous epithelium and is also seen in some neoplasms. In hyperplasia the ratio of nucleus to cytoplasm is normal.

Approaching the MCQ paper

You are allowed 3 hours to complete 90 multiple choice questions. There are 30 questions in each of the disciplines of anatomy, physiology and pathology. The questions are all of the same format as those in this book. There is a statement called a stem followed by five responses marked a, b, c, d and e. Read each response together with the stem and decide whether the whole statement is true or false. Mark your answer on the answer grid provided or on the question paper itself. If you take the latter course you must allow enough time at the end to transfer your answers on to the grid. The examiners are very strict and will not allow you to run over time, even if you are merely transferring the answers! Each response should be treated separately from the other responses in the same question. This means that any combination of true and false answers is possible, ranging from all true to all false. If you have no idea what the answer is you are allowed to answer 'don't know'. However, our advise is that you make an attempt by playing your hunches. This is not the same as pure guesswork.

In marking the paper, 1 point is scored if your answer (true or false) is correct and 1 point is deducted if incorrect. Obviously no credit is given and none is taken away for a 'don't know'.

The questions in this book are modelled on actual FRCS questions. In our experience of the examination we have found that some questions are badly worded and some contain significant spelling mistakes. Such errors are usually weeded out by the next set of examiners, but this is no guarantee of perfect MCQs.

Our questions are aimed as tests of your knowledge and as stimuli to further reading. The explanations to the answers are full when the question is tackling a tricky subject and brief when we feel the answers are relatively straightforward.

Practice examination paper

Questions

1. **In the middle ear—**
   a. The superior bulb of the internal jugular vein lies beneath the floor
   b. The roof is formed by the tegmen tympani
   c. The internal carotid artery lies anteriorly
   d. The auditory tube enters through the anterior wall
   e. It is in communication with the mastoid antrum posteriorly

2. **Muscles of mastication—**
   a. The medial pterygoid retracts the jaw
   b. The lateral pterygoid arises in part from the maxillary tubercle
   c. The temporalis muscle arise from the temporal fossa between the superior temporal line and the infratemporal crest
   d. The digastric muscles are important in opening the mouth
   e. The masseter is supplied by a branch of the anterior division of the mandibular nerve

3. **The following structures are derived from tissue of the second branchial arch—**
   a. Posterior third of tongue
   b. The incus and stapes
   c. The maxillary artery
   d. The stylohyoid ligament
   e. The stylohyoid muscle

4. **The vagus nerve—**
   a. Emerges from the brain between the pyramid and the inferior olive
   b. Contains motor fibres, which originate in the nucleus ambiguus
   c. Contributes to the pharyngeal plexus
   d. Innervates the stylopharyngeus muscle
   e. Gives off the superior laryngeal branch from the superior ganglion

5. **The tongue—**
   a. Develops in the roof of the primitive pharynx
   b. Is supplied by the glossopharyngeal nerve in its posterior two-thirds
   c. Deviates to the right when protruded, if the right hypoglossal nerve is damaged
   d. Contains a muscle supplied by the pharyngeal plexus
   e. Is the site of origin of the thymus gland

6. **In the neck—**
   a. The phrenic nerve runs from medial to lateral across the scalenus anterior muscle
   b. The dorsal scapular nerve runs through scalenus medius
   c. The middle sympathetic cervical ganglion lies at C6
   d. The facial artery arises from the external carotid artery above the lingual artery
   e. The inferior thyroid artery arises from the costocervical trunk of the subclavian artery

7. **Considering the posterior belly of digastric—**
   a. The hypoglossal nerve runs anteriorly
   b. The internal jugular vein runs posteriorly
   c. The lingual artery runs posteriorly
   d. It arises on the medial side of the mastoid process
   e. It is supplied by a branch of the facial nerve

8. **The radial nerve—**
   a. Originates from the medial cord of the brachial plexus
   b. Gives off branches to the long, medial and short heads of triceps in the axilla
   c. Accompanies the profunda brachii artery in the spiral groove
   d. Supplies part of the brachialis muscle
   e. Emerges between the brachioradialis and extensor carpi radialis longus

9. **Concerning the humerus—**
   a. The head is at the growing end
   b. Subscapularis inserts on to the lesser tubercle (tuberosity)
   c. The medial head of triceps arises from above the spiral groove
   d. The presence of a supratrochlear spur may explain symptoms of ulnar nerve palsy
   e. Fracture of the surgical neck may lead to paralysis of the deltoid muscle

10. **The clavicle—**
    a. Develops in membrane
    b. Is the first bone of the skeleton to develop
    c. Gives a tendinous origin to sternocleidomastoid from its medial third
    d. The sternoclavicular joint is an atypical synovial joint
    e. Gives origin to part of sternothyroid

11. **Regarding the axilla—**
    a. The medial side of the first rib forms a medial boundary
    b. The axillary vein is lateral to the axillary artery
    c. It contains the divisions of the brachial plexus
    d. The lateral group of lymph nodes drain the arm
    e. The musculocutaneous nerve arises from the medial cord of the brachial plexus

12. **In the hand—**
    a. The superficial palmar arch is nearly always complete
    b. The radial artery enters the palm by passing between the two heads of opponens pollicis
    c. The transverse head of the adductor pollicis arises from the base of the second and third metacarpals
    d. The lateral side of the forefinger is supplied by the ulnar artery
    e. There is more abduction than adduction at the wrist joint

13. Vasculature of the abdomen—
- a. Branches of the splenic artery enter the hilum separately
- b. The inferior pancreaticoduodenal artery is a branch of the gastroduodenal artery
- c. The left lumbar veins pass posterior to the aorta
- d. Venous blood from the head of the pancreas usually drains into the splenic vein
- e. The left suprarenal vein is shorter than the right

14. Regarding the duodenum—
- a. The first part is longer in males
- b. The hepatic flexure lies superiorly to the second part
- c. The superior mesenteric artery passes posteriorly
- d. Histologically it has characteristic Brunner's glands
- e. The inferior mesenteric vein is lateral to the fourth part

15. The pancreas—
- a. Has a head, which lies on the transpyloric plane
- b. Has a tail, which lies in the lienorenal ligament
- c. Has a uncinate process, which is derived from the ventral pancreatic bud
- d. Has the main duct of Santorini, which may open with the common bile duct into the second part of the duodenum
- e. Has a neck, which lies in front of the origin of the portal vein and the superior mesenteric artery

16. The transpyloric plane—
- a. Marks the level of the head of the pancreas
- b. Marks the level of the fundus of the gallbladder
- c. Marks the level of the seventh costal cartilage
- d. Marks the origin of the hepatic portal vein, which is formed by the union of the superior mesenteric vein with the splenic vein
- e. Marks the termination of the spinal cord

17. The inguinal canal—
- a. Has the lacunar ligament as part of its floor
- b. Has a posterior wall formed partly by the conjoint tendon
- c. Is about 10 cm long
- d. Has a superficial ring, which lies directly anterior to the deep ring in the baby
- e. Has the inferior epigastric vessels lying along the lateral wall of the deep ring

18. At cholecystectomy—
  a. The gall bladder overlies part of the duodenum
  b. Ligation of the cystic artery cuts off all arterial blood supply to the gall bladder
  c. The cystic artery may be derived from a branch of the superior mesenteric artery
  d. The gall bladder may be dependent from a mesentery
  e. Accidental ligation of the right hepatic artery causes infarction of the quadrate lobe

19. The urinary bladder—
  a. Is lined by transitional epithelium containing mucous glands
  b. Is supplied in part with blood derived from the external iliac artery
  c. Has a lymphatic drainage to both the internal and external iliac nodes
  d. Is formed from the lower part of the urogenital sinus
  e. Has a trigone which, in the male, overlies the median lobe of the prostate

20. The pelvis—
  a. The epoophoron and paraoophoron in the female are remnants of the paramesonephric system
  b. The levator ani arises partly from the fascia covering obturator externus
  c. The prostate consists of acini embedded in a connective tissue stroma
  d. The vagina is partly covered anteriorly by peritoneum
  e. Lymph from the body of the uterus may drain to the inguinal nodes

21. Regarding the sciatic nerve—
  a. It is endangered by an intramuscular injection in the upper outer quadrant of the buttock
  b. Its common peroneal branch may emerge above piriformis
  c. It supplies part of adductor longus
  d. It is supplied by a remnant of the original axial artery of the lower limb
  e. It lies on the tendon of obturator externus

22. **As regards the talus—**
    a. It has an aponeurotic attachment from tibialis posterior
    b. Flexor hallucis longus tendon passes between the medial and lateral tubercles of the posterior process
    c. It is wider in front
    d. The lateral articular facet is smaller than the medial
    e. Part of the posterior process may be separate in 5% of cases

23. **The knee joint—**
    a. The medial facet of the patella is in contact with the femur in extension
    b. The posterior cruciate ligament is intrasynovial
    c. The medial collateral ligament is attached to the medial menisucs
    d. The anterior cruciate attaches to the medial femoral condyle
    e. In locking of the knee in extension the femur rotates laterally on the tibia

24. **Concerning the femoral triangle—**
    a. Its lateral boundary is the medial border of sartorius
    b. It contains the nerve to vastus medialis
    c. The profunda femoris artery emerges medial to the common femoral artery
    d. The femoral vein passes anterior to the superficial femoral artery
    e. Adductor longus forms the medial wall

25. **The following medially rotate the hip—**
    a. Gluteus medius
    b. Gluteus maximus
    c. Adductor longus
    d. Iliacus
    e. Quadratus femorus

26. **The oesophagus—**
    a. Is 15 cm long
    b. Is a posterior relation of the left atrium
    c. Lies anterior to part of the descending aorta
    d. Is partially supplied by the recurrent laryngeal nerve
    e. Is constricted by the right main bronchus

27. **A computed tomography scan of the body at the level of the sternal angle (of Louis) will show—**
   a. The intervertebral disc between T4 and T5
   b. The azygous vein
   c. Part of the lower lobe of the lung on each side
   d. The sympathetic chain
   e. The bifurcation of the pulmonary trunk

28. **The heart—**
   a. Has the right atrium in which the posterior wall is smooth and which is derived from the right sinus venosus
   b. Has a base, which is mainly formed by the left atrium
   c. Contains musculi pectinati in the ventricles
   d. Contains the coronary sinus, which drains into the left atrium
   e. Contains the sinoatrial node, which is situated just to the left of the superior vena cava

29. **In the lungs—**
   a. The surface marking of the oblique fissure is the lateral border of the scapula in a fully abducted arm
   b. The sympathetic nerve supply is shared with the heart
   c. The bronchi are supplied directly from the aorta
   d. The pulmonary artery lies in the lowest part of the hilum
   e. The course of the pulmonary veins closely follows the bronchial tree

30. **Embryologically—**
   a. The medial umbilical ligament is derived from the obliterated umbilical artery
   b. The aortic arch is formed from the left third arch artery
   c. the ventral pancreatic bud forms the uncinate process
   d. The midgut herniates (physiological umbilical herniation) at about 6 weeks
   e. The third pharyngeal pouch gives rise to the thymus and to the inferior parathyroid gland

31. The following are characteristic of smooth muscle—
   a. It contain striations
   b. It has a poorly developed sarcoplasmic reticulum
   c. It may contract spontaneously independent of its nerve supply
   d. It contains less actin and myosin than skeletal muscle
   e. It relies heavily on the Krebs cycle for energy

32. The following are cutaneous sensory organs—
   a. Merkel's discs
   b. Meissner's plexus
   c. Naked nerve endings
   d. Dense core vesicles
   e. Ruffini endings

33. In a stretch reflex such as the knee jerk—
   a. The pathway of the reflex arc is monosynaptic
   b. The receptor for the reflex is the Golgi tendon organ
   c. Stimulation of gamma efferents leads directly to the contraction of extrafusal fibres
   d. Central delay accounts for 0.3 s of the reflex time
   e. The law of Bell–Magendie is obeyed

34. After denervation of a skeletal muscle—
   a. The area of muscle sensitive to acetylcholine decreases
   b. The number of muscle acetylcholine receptors may increase
   c. Muscle fibres show Wallerian degeneration
   d. Strong electrical stimulation of the muscle delays atrophy
   e. The muscle tends to lengthen if physiotherapy is not undertaken

35. In considering the pathophysiology of cerebrospinal fluid—
   a. Normal lumbar pressure is 70–180 mm of cerebrospinal fluid
   b. Absorption by the arachnoid villi is independent of pressure
   c. Cerebrospinal fluid from the fourth ventricle flows into the cisterna magna
   d. The headache following post lumbar puncture can be relieved by an intrathecal injection of sterile isotonic saline
   e. In communicating hydrocephalus, fluid flows readily from the ventricular system into the subarachnoid space

36. **In the adult human ear—**
    a. The tympanic membrane stops vibrating almost immediately after the sound wave stops
    b. The tympanic reflex is effective in protecting against sound from a sudden gunshot
    c. The range of audible sound is 20–20 000 kHz
    d. Response to caloric stimulation depends on convection currents causing movement of the basilar membrane
    e. The Schwabach test demonstrates the phenomenon of masking

37. **Excitatory neurotransmitters, which are found in the central nervous system, include—**
    a. Glycine
    b. Gamma-aminobutyric acid
    c. Aspartate
    d. Dopamine
    e. Glutamate

38. **Concerning cardiac output—**
    a. It may increase to 20 l/min in the trained athlete without an increase in autonomic stimulation
    b. The average venous return to the right atrium is 5 l/min
    c. It may be increased by an arteriovenous fistula
    d. It increases significantly when the mean systemic filling pressure is 14 mmHg
    e. When measured by the Fick principle, it requires a knowledge of oxygen consumption, heart rate and blood pressure

39. **In the electrocardiogram—**
    a. The normal PR interval is 0.12–0.20 s
    b. The PR interval increases in atrioventricular nodal block
    c. The duration of the QRS complex may be greater than 0.12 s in left bundle branch block
    d. The ST interval represents ventricular repolarization
    e. Digoxin may cause T-wave inversion

40. During exercise—

  a. There is a gradual increase in ventilation rate at the onset of moderate exercise

  b. The metabolic rate of muscle may increase up to 100-fold

  c. The respiratory quotient is greater than 1.5 if the exercise is strenuous

  d. Blood pH rises due to anaerobic work

  e. Cardiac output may increase 10-fold

41. In the cardiac cycle—

  a. The first heart sound corresponds to the closure of the atrioventricular valves when the pressure in the ventricles exceeds that in the atria

  b. Isometric ventricular relaxation begins when the aortic valve opens

  c. The ventricle normally ejects about 120 ml of blood during each contraction

  d. The diastolic phase of the cycle shortens more markedly than the systolic phase during exercise

  e. The C wave of the venous pulsations corresponds to bulging of the tricuspid valve during ventricular contraction

42. In control of the blood pressure—

  a. The central nervous system ischaemic receptor provides a powerful response but only at a blood pressure of less than 60 mmHg

  b. The main baroreceptor site in humans is in the aortic arch

  c. The baroreceptor is stimulated by a rise in the intraarterial pressure

  d. Low-pressure receptors in the atria and great vessels are stimulated by decrease in the volume of the right atrium and great veins

  e. The heart normally has a resting vagal tone

43. The compliance of the lungs—

  a. Is a measure of the pressure–volume relationship of the lungs

  b. Is decreased in emphysema

  c. Is decreased in pulmonary fibrosis

  d. Is increased in pulmonary congestion

  e. Is half the value if one lung is removed

44. The effects of gravity on the circulation include—
  a. Reduction of the central blood pool by as much as 400 ml
  b. Reduction of cardiac output by 25%
  c. Reduction of the stroke volume by as much as 40%
  d. Increase in the leg volume by as much as 600 ml
  e. Increase in the total peripheral resistance by 25%

45. Osteoporosis—
  a. Results from an imbalance between bone resorption and formation affecting mainly cortical bone
  b. Is significantly more common in women than men
  c. Is associated with both hyperthyroidism and hyperparathyroidism
  d. Shows minimal or no derangement of bone biochemistry
  e. May be treated by the biphosphonates which inhibit bone resorption

46. Concerning analgesics—
  a. Aspirin inhibits the lipoxygenase enzyme during prostaglandin synthesis
  b. Codeine is a semisynthetic drug
  c. Paracetamol has a mild anti-inflammatory action
  d. Morphine is a natural alkaloid acting on μ opioid receptors
  e. Naloxone antagonizes all opiate effects

47. The following drugs are positively inotropic—
  a. Nifedipine
  b. Dopamine
  c. Theophylline
  d. Glucagon
  e. Adenosine

48. In spermatogenesis—
  a. The Leydig cells are important in supporting and nourishing the spermatozoa
  b. Inhibin secretion corresponds to the rate of spermatogenesis
  c. Testosterone increases the secretion of luteinizing hormone
  d. Testosterone is required to initiate spermatogenesis
  e. Inhibin is secreted by Leydig cells

49. In the human menstrual cycle—
  a. Follicle-stimulating hormone is mainly responsble for follicular development and oestradiol secretion
  b. Oestradiol at low concentration depresses follicle-stimulating hormone secretion
  c. Oestradiol at high concentration is responsible for the midcycle luteinizing hormone
  d. Progesterone at high concentration produces a positive feedback effect on luteinizing hormone
  e. Oestradiol and progesterone probably mediate their effects by altering the sensitivity of the pituitary gland to gonadotrophin-releasing hormone

50. The following statements about renal tubular function are true—
  a. Some 40–50% of sodium in the glomerular filtrate is reabsorbed in the proximal tubule
  b. Potassium and hydrogen are secreted into the glomerular filtrate at some point along the tubule
  c. Sodium is the principal ion reabsorbed in the diluting segment of the early distal tubule
  d. Passive diffusion of large amounts of urea from the collecting duct contributes to the marked increase in the osmolality of the medullary interstitial fluid
  e. The countercurrent exchange system of the vasa recta is essential for the formation of a concentrated urine

51. The kidney—
  a. Contains about 1 million nephrons in humans
  b. Contains principal cells in the collecting ducts which respond to antidiuretic hormone
  c. Contains intercalated cells in the collecting duct which secrete acid
  d. Contains vasa recta which are low-resistance vessels
  e. Synthesizes 1,25 dihydroxyvitamin D

52. Normal growth requirements include—
  a. A diet adequate in calories
  b. Thyroid hormones
  c. Insulin
  d. Androgens
  e. Oestrogens

53. **The following mechanisms are involved in preventing the breakdown of proteins in starvation—**
    a. Formation of ketone bodies
    b. Conversion of thryoxine to triiodothyronine
    c. Protection of glucose by cortisol
    d. Deamination and gluconeogenesis in the kidney
    e. The use of ketones by the brain and kidney as a source of energy

54. **In the period immediately after severe trauma—**
    a. There is an increase in the level of plasma free fatty acids and glycerol
    b. There is an increase in body temperature
    c. There is an increase in oxygen consumption
    d. There is a decrease in cell membrane potential
    e. Glucose tolerance is increased

55. **Considering the thyroid hormones—**
    a. Triiodothyronine binds to cell membrane receptors
    b. They increase the number of beta-adrenergic receptors in the heart
    c. Cholesterol levels increase in hyperthyroidism
    d. Most of the circulating thyroxine is bound to albumin
    e. They shift the oxygen haemoglobin dissociation curve to the right

56. **The following increase gastrointestinal motility—**
    a. Gastrin
    b. 5-Hydroxytryptamine
    c. Secretin
    d. Substance P
    e. Adrenaline

57. **After total hepatectomy—**
    a. The blood urea rises
    b. The blood ammonia rises
    c. Hypoglycaemia is common
    d. There is little effect on the plasma protein level
    e. There is marked hypogammaglobulinaemia

58. In the colon—
a. Mass action contraction plays a major part in the propulsion of chyme
b. Sodium is reabsorbed followed by water
c. Water-soluble vitamins are absorbed
d. The frequency of the slow wave increases from proximal to distal
e. The mucosa contains crypts of Lieberkühn, lined almost entirely by goblet cells

59. Gastric secretions include—
a. Hydrochloric acid from the chief cells
b. Pepsinogens secreted by the parietal cells
c. Intrinsic factor secreted by parietal cells
d. Gastrin secreted by the parietal cells in the antrum
e. Amylase secreted by the chief cells

60. Concerning pancreatic secretion—
a. At low flow rates, the anion is mainly chloride
b. It contains sodium and potassium ions at approximately the same concentration as in plasma at all flow rates
c. It is stimulated by secretin, which only has effects on the inorganic fraction
d. It is stimulated by gastrin, which has effects on the organic as well as potentiating the effects of secretin
e. It contains proteolytic enzyme precursors

61. The following show multifactorial inheritance—
a. Pyrloric stenosis
b. Congenital dislocation of the hip
c. Classical haemophilia
d. Familial polyposis coli
e. Congenital adrenal hyperplasia

62. Human leukocyte antigens—
a. Are coded in humans by genes located in the short arm of chromosome 6
b. Are found on red cells
c. Play an important part in antigen recognition by B cells
d. Show variation between ethnic groups
e. In humans at loci A and B code for class 1 molecules

63. Haemochromatosis—
a. Causes skin pigmentation as a result of melanin
b. Is an autosomal recessive condition
c. Has an increased risk of primary carcinoma of the liver
d. Affects women more than men
e. Deposition of iron in the spleen leads to the term 'sago' spleen

64. In osteoarthrosis—
a. There is fibrillation of the cartilage surface
b. There is proliferation of fibroblasts and formation of a pannus
c. X-rays reveal subchondral cysts
d. Osteophytes are a recognized feature
e. There is marked synovial proliferation

65. Concerning adult respiratory distress syndrome—
a. Sepsis is a major cause
b. Pulmonary oedema of cardiac cause is characteristic
c. It may present with refractory hypoxaemia
d. It is commonly complicated by secondary pulmonary infection with resistant organisms
e. It is readily treated with steroids

66. Subacute bacterial endocarditis—
a. Usually affects normal hearts
b. Rarely has extracardiac foci
c. Is associated with low-virulence organisms
d. Most commonly affects the aortic valve
e. May produce severe valvular distortion

67. Myasthenia gravis—
a. May be associated with a thymic neoplasm
b. May be associated with thymic hyperplasia
c. Involves immunoglobulin M antibodies to the nicotinic acetylcholine receptor
d. With superimposed infection may precipitate a mysasthenic crisis
e. Is a rare non-metastatic manifestation of oat cell carcinoma of the lung

68. Considering candidiasis—
   a. *Candida albicans* is a non-sporing bacterium
   b. Broad-spectrum antibiotics are useful in the treatment of candidiasis
   c. In a healthy individual, large numbers of *Candida albicans* are found in the mouth and bowel
   d. *Candida* infection is more commen when the blood sugar level is poorly controlled
   e. *Candida* is a cause of intertrigo in the submammary folds

69. Considering gas gangrene—
   a. There is necrosis with putrefaction
   b. Treatment with low-dose penicillin is indicated
   c. The causative agents include *Clostridium perfringens* and *C. oedematiens*
   d. Treatment with hyperbaric oxygen is useful
   e. The infective agents can be detected on the perineal skin of healthy subjects

70. The following viruses produce latent infections—
   a. Mumps virus
   b. Herpes simplex virus type 1
   c. Coxsackievirus
   d. Varicella-zoster virus
   e. Influenza virus

71. Hepatitis infection—
   a. May be caused by the DNA-containing hepatitis A virus
   b. Caused by hepatitis A virus is transmitted by the faeco-oral route
   c. Caused by hepatitis A virus may lead to cirrhosis of the liver
   d. In the presence of the HBe antigen in the serum correlates with high infectivity
   e. In the presence of the HBc antigen correlates with high infectivity

72. Actinomyces israelii—
a. Exists as a saprophyte in the mouth and in the alimentary tract
b. Produces cervicofacial abscesses
c. Spreads via lymphatics
d. Produces pus which contains sulphur granules
e. Is a microaerophilic organism

73. Wasserman antibodies (anticardiolipin) are found in—
a. Malaria
b. Leprosy
c. Trypanosomiasis
d. Systemic lupus erythematosus
e. Glandular fever

74. Exotoxins—
a. Are predominantly lipid in form
b. Are heat-stable
c. Exert non-specific affects on a variety of tissues
d. Are of high potency
e. Are commonly produced by *clostridia*

75. Hypokalaemia may be associated with
a. Metabolic acidosis
b. The use of carbonic anhydrase inhibitors
c. Pyloric stenosis
d. Secondary hyperaldosteronism
e. Villous papilloma of the large bowel

76. In pyloric stenosis—
a. There is hyperkalaemic alkalosis
b. There is hyponatraemia
c. An acid urine is excreted in the advanced cases
d. The total calcium concentration falls
e. Urea concentration falls due to vomiting

77. Albumin—
   a. Has a molecular weight of 65 000
   b. Has a half-life of 10 days
   c. Is present at a lower concentration in the plasma compartment compared with the interstitial compartment
   d. Levels are unaffected by the process of acute inflammation
   e. May be lost from the skin in diseases such as psoriasis

78. B-lymphocytes—
   a. Differentiate into plasma cells
   b. Are infected by the human immunodeficiency virus
   c. Form rosettes with sheep red blood cells
   d. Have Fc receptors on their surface
   e. Have C3b receptors on their surface

79. Macrocytosis is found in—
   a. Hyperthyroidism
   b. Pernicious anaemia
   c. Treatment with anticonvulsants
   d. Aplastic anaemia
   e. Hereditary spherocytosis

80. Platelets—
   a. Have a present but indistinct nucleus
   b. Have a mean life span of 7–10 days
   c. Contain 5-hydroxytryptamine
   d. Possess a poorly developed canalicular system on their surface
   e. Function is unaffected in von Willebrand's disease

81. Concerning diseases of the breast—
   a. Pericanalicular fibroadenomas predominate in young women
   b. Family history is an important aetiological factor in ductal carcinoma
   c. There is a 40–50% chance of lobular carcinoma being bilateral
   d. The degree of lymphocytic response to a tumour has no bearing on the prognosis
   e. Intralobular carcinoma is commoner than intraductal

82. **Sites which may undergo metaplasia include—**
    a. Bronchus
    b. Prostate
    c. Bladder
    d. Gall bladder
    e. Stomach

83. **In multiple myeloma—**
    a. M proteins are found in the serum
    b. There is a neoplastic proliferation of T cells
    c. In most cases immunoglobulin G is the immunoglobulin produced
    d. Bence Jones proteins redissolve when the urine is heated to 70°C
    e. There may be hypocalcaemia

84. **Considering oesophageal neoplasms—**
    a. Adenocarcinoma is usually found in the lower third
    b. Tylosis is a predisposing factor
    c. Carcinoma-*in-situ* may be found
    d. The commonest benign tumour is the squamous papilloma
    e. Chagas disease (South American trypanosomiasis) predisposes to carcinoma

85. **Adenocarcinoma of the prostate gland—**
    a. Typically causes osteoblastic bone lesions
    b. Typically causes osteoclastic bone lesions
    c. Is a common finding at autopsy of patients over 80 years of age
    d. Is testosterone-dependent
    e. Produces elevated plasma acid phosphatase levels only if metastasis occurs

86. **The following factors affect healing—**
    a. Zinc therapy when the serum level is normal
    b. Infection
    c. Increasing the normal room temperature by 10°C
    d. Ionizing radiation
    e. Diet

87. The following statements are true of the level of C-reactive protein
   a. It is raised in pneumococcal pneumonia
   b. It is raised in rheumatoid arthritis
   c. It is decreased in trauma
   d. It usually varies inversely with the erythrocyte sedimentation rate
   e. It decreases by 50% per day if antibiotic treatment is successful

88. In the process of wound contraction—
   a. Myoepithelial cells approximate the wound edges
   b. Collagen contraction plays a role
   c. Vitamin C deficiency is detrimental
   d. Immediate skin grafting prevents further contraction
   e. Wound size may be reduced by up to 80% of its original size

89. Papillary necrosis is caused by—
   a. Chronic ingestion of aspirin
   b. Sickle cell anaemia
   c. Diabetes insipidus
   d. Alcoholism
   e. Beta-thalassaemia

90. Neutrophils—
   a. Have segmented nuclei and granular cytoplasm
   b. Contain lactoferrin, an iron-binding agent
   c. Use glucose as energy via the Embden–Meyerhof pathway
   d. Show failure of lysosomal fusion in Chediak–Higashi syndrome
   e. Synthesis may be inhibited by chloramphenicol

Answers

1. All
The middle ear is an air-conditioning cavity in the petrous part of a temporal bone. The floor is usually a thin piece of bone which may be deficient but may also be fibrous in nature. The tegmen tympani is part of the petrous temporal bone and separates the middle ear from the meninges. The canal for the tensor tympani muscle also lies in the anterior wall. The large opening to the mastoid is called the aditus.

2. d. e.
There are five muscles of mastication: the medial pterygoid closes and protracts the jaw as well as moving it medially. The lateral pterygoid arises from the infratemporal surface of the skull and the lateral surface of the lateral pterygoid plate. The medial pterygoid arises from the medial side of the medial pterygoid plate as well as from the maxillary tubercle. The temporalis muscle arises from the temporal fossa between the inferior temporal line and infratemporal crest. The temporalis fascia arises from superior temporal line.

3. d. e.
The posterior third of the tongue is derived from the third arch. The incus and part of the maxillary artery are first arch structures. The stapes, stylohyoid ligament and stylohyoid muscle are second arch structures.

4. b. c.
The vagus nerve emerges from the brain between the inferior olive and the inferior cerebellar peduncle.
  Stylopharyngeus muscle is supplied by the glossopharyngeal nerve.
  The superior laryngeal nerve comes off the vagus nerve at the inferior ganglion.

5. c. d.
The tongue develops in the floor of the mouth and is supplied with common sensation by the lingual nerve (anterior two-thirds) and glossopharyngeal nerve (posterior third). The tongue muscles are all supplied by the hypoglossal nerve except for palatoglossus, which is supplied by the pharnygeal plexus. If the hypoglossal nerve is damaged the tongue deviates towards the damaged side. The thymus originates from the third pharyngeal pouch, whereas the thyroid develops from the foramen caecum of the tongue.

6. b. c. d.
The phrenic nerve runs laterally to medially across the scalenus anterior beneath the prevertebral fascia. The inferior thyroid artery arises from the thyrocervical trunk, which is a branch of the first part of the subclavian artery.

7. b. c. d. e.
The posterior belly of digastric arises from the digastric notch on the medial side of the mastoid process. It is joined to the anterior belly by an intermediate tendon which passes through a sling which is attached to the hyoid bone. The hypoglossal nerve runs posteriorly.

8. c. d.
The radial nerve originates from the posterior cord. It gives off branches to the long and medial heads of triceps only in the axilla. The radial nerve emerges between the brachialis and brachioradialis muscles.

9. a. b. e.
The head of the humerus and the distal end of the femur are at the growing ends ('from the knee I flee to the elbow I grow'). The medial head of triceps arises from the humeral shaft below the spiral groove. The supratrochlear spur is associated with the ligament of Struthers, which connects the spur to the medial epicondyle. The median nerve and/or the brachial artery may pass under the ligament and lead to median nerve palsy or ischaemic symptoms in the hand. Fracture of the surgical neck may damage the axillary nerve which supplies deltoid.

10. a. b.
The clavicle is the first bone of the skeleton to develop, usually beginning to ossify at 5 weeks *in utero*. It develops in membrane before any cartilage is present in the fetus. Its medial third gives a muscular origin to sternocleidomastoid. The sternoclavicular joint is an atypical synovial joint as both of the bone ends are covered with fibrocartilage and there is a fibrocartilaginous disc separating the joint into two cavities. The origin of sternohyoid encroaches upon the posterior surface of the clavicle.

11. d.
The axilla is a pyramidal space allowing the neurovasculature and lymphatics to pass between the neck and arms. The medial border of the axilla contains the upper part of serratus anterior and ribs; however it is the lateral border of the first rib which forms part of this boundary. The axillary vein is formed from the venae comitantes of the brachial artery and basilic vein, and it lies medial to the axillary artery. The trunks of the brachial plexus are found in the posterior triangle of the neck, the divisions behind the clavicle and the cords within the axilla. The musculocutaneous nerve arises from the lateral cord of the plexus.

12. None
In two-thirds of cases the superficial palmar arch is not complete. When it is, it communicates with the superficial branch of the radial artery. The radial artery enters the hand by passing through the first dorsal interosseous and between the two heads of adductor pollicis. The transverse head of adductor pollicis arises from the third metacarpal with the oblique head arising from the base of the second and third metacarpal and adjacent carpal bones. The lateral side of the forefinger is supplied by the radialis indicis artery, a branch of the radial artery. The radial styloid projects more distally than the ulnar styloid and hence there is more adduction than abduction at the wrist joint.

13. a. c.
The tortuous splenic artery, passing in or above the pancreas, runs in the lienorenal ligament and enters the hilum as separate branches. The inferior pancreaticoduodenal artery is a branch of the superior mesenteric artery and so supplies the commencement of the midgut from below the entrance of the bile duct as well as the head of the pancreas. The left lumbar veins pass behind the aorta and are in danger of rupture when mobilizing the aorta during aneurysm repair. Venous blood from the head of the pancreas usually drains via the superior and inferior pancreaticoduodenal veins, which enter the portal vein and superior mesenteric vein respectively. The right suprarenal vein enters the inferior vena cava and is very short.

14.   b. d. e.
The duodenum is C-shaped and 25 cm long. Descriptively it is divided into four parts. The first part is intraperitoneal, longer in females than males and is closely related to the gall bladder. The second and third part are both retroperitoneal. The second part lies on the hilum of the right kidney with the head of the pancreas and common bile duct related medially. It is also closely related to the hepatic flexure. The third part lies on the right psoas, inferior vena cava and aorta. Important anterior relations are the superior mesenteric vessels. The fourth part is medial to the inferior mesenteric vein. Brunner's glands, which are characteristic, are branched and twirled and lie beneath the muscularis mucosae.

15.   b. c. e.
The neck of the pancreas lies on the transpyloric plane (L1).

The main pancreatic duct is the duct of Wirsung. The duct of Santorini is the accessory pancreatic duct.

16.   b. d. e.
It is the neck of the pancreas which lies at the level of the transpyloric plane. The origin of the hepatic portal vein lies behind the neck of the pancreas. The head of the pancreas lies below the transpyloric plane. It is the ninth costal cartilage, not the seventh, which lies at the level of the transpyloric plane. This point intersects with the hiatus semilunaris, which marks the lateral margin of the rectus abdominis muscle. This point also marks the fundus of the gall bladder on the right side.

17.   a. b. d.
The inguinal canal is about 4 cm long.

The inferior epigatric vessels lie along the medial wall of the deep ring. They demarcate the direct inguinal hernia, which passes medial to these vessels from an indirect inguinal hernia, which passes lateral to these vessels.

18.   a. c. d.
The gall bladder overlies the junction of the first and second parts of the duodenum. It receives blood from both the cystic artery and gall bladder bed. The cystic artery is usually a branch of the right hepatic artery which may be derived from the superior mesenteric

artery. On occasion the gall bladder hangs on a mesentery, at which torsion is possible. The right hepatic artery does not usually supply the quadrate lobe.

19. b. c. e.
The bladder epithelium contains no glands. The pubic branch of the inferior epigastric artery (a branch of the external iliac artery) sends twigs which supply the bladder. The bladder is derived from the superior part of the urogenital sinus. In the male, the median lobe may project above the internal urethral orifice as the uvula vesicae. This projects into the trigone.

20. e.
The fallopian tubes, uterus and upper vagina develop from the paramesonephric system. The epoophoron and paraoophoron are remnants of the mesonephric system. The levator ani partly arises from the fascia on obturator internus. Histologically, the prostate is characterized by acini being embedded in a fibromuscular stroma. Anteriorly the peritoneum does not extend down as far as the vagina; however, posteriorly it extends down to cover the posterior fornix. Lymph from the body of the uterus usually drains to the external iliac nodes but may drain to the inguinal nodes by the round ligament.

21. b. d.
The common peroneal division may emerge above (0.5%), through (12%) or below piriformis. The sciatic nerve supplies part of adductor magnus and lies on the tendon of obturator internus. The nerve is supplied partly by the arteria comitans nervi ischiadici, the remnant of the original axial artery.

22. b. e.
The talus carries the whole body weight but has no muscle attachments. It is wider in front than it is behind so that there is less inversion and eversion in dorsiflexion than there is in plantar flexion. The lateral tubercle on the posterior process may be separate in 5% of cases – the so-called os trigonum.

23. c.
The medial facet of the patella is in contact with the femur in

flexion. The cruciate ligaments are intracapsuler but extrasynovial. The anterior cruciate ligament attaches to the lateral femoral condyle, with the posterior cruciate being attached to the medial femoral condyle. In locking of the knee, the femur rotates medially on the tibial plateau: the reverse occurs to unlock the knee.

24. a. b. e.
The base of the triangle is the inguinal ligament. Its medial boundary is the medial border of adductor longus and its lateral boundary is the medial border of sartorius. It contains the nerve to vastus medialis and the saphenous nerve. The femoral vein passes deep to the superficial femoral artery and profunda femoris usually emerges posterolaterally to the common femoral artery. The floor of the triangle is formed by iliacus, pectineus and adductor longus.

25. a. c. d.
Lateral rotators of the hip are those muscles which pass obliquely or transversely across the back of the hip joint. These include the gluteus maximus, piriformis, obturator internus, the gemelli and the quadratus femoris. Posterior fibres of gluteus medius and gluteus minimus may also cause lateral rotation. Similarly, any muscle which passes in front of the hip joint causes medial rotation. These include gluteus medius and gluteus minimus, as well as psoas major, iliacus, pectineus and adductor longus.

26. b. c. d.
The oesophagus is a muscular tube which extends from the cricoid cartilage at C6 down as far as the cardia of the stomach. It is 25 cm long. The upper third of the oesophagus is said to contain striated muscle whereas the bottom two-thirds is said to contain visceral muscle. Thus the recurrent larygngeal nerve supplies the upper part, the rest being supplied by the autonomic system. The left main bronchus may constrict the oesophagus, as may the left atrium when enlarged.

27. a. b. c. d.
The angle of Louis and manubriosternal joint are synonymous. At this level the azygous vein is seen entering the superior vena cava and the trachea bifurcates. The apical segment of each lower lobe is visible as a crescentic area in the posterior part of each pleural

cavity. The bifurcation of the pulmonary trunk is at T5.

28. a. b.

Musculi pectinati are found in the atria of the heart.

The coronary sinus drains into the right atrium, not into the left.

The sinoatrial node is situated just to the right of the superior vena cava.

29. c.

It is the medial (vertebral) border of the scapula in an abducted arm which marks the oblique fissure. The sympathetic supply to the heart is from the cardiac branches of the cervical ganglia whereas the lung is supplied from the upper four thoracic ganglia. The pulmonary veins lie lowest in the hilum and are thus able to expand between the leaves of the pulmonary ligament. Every bronchus is accompanied by a branch of the pulmonary artery, but the pulmonary veins pass in the intersegmental septa.

30. a. c. d. e.

The aortic arch is derived from the left fourth arch artery. The left third arch artery gives rise to the left common carotid artery.

31. b. c. d.

A smooth muscle differs from skeletal muscle in that it does not have the characteristic striated pattern. It has a poorly developed sarcoplasmic reticulum; however there may be scattered vesicles, which function as calcium stores. It may be referred to as involuntary muscle, as it may contract spontaneously or in response to autonomic stimulation. Contractile filaments of actin and myosin are present in smooth muscle but there is only 10% of the amount present in skeletal muscle. Smooth muscle has few mitochondria and hence relies mainly on glycolysis for its metabolic needs.

32. a. c. e.

Meissner's corpuscles are sensory endings but the plexus is in the intestinal wall. Dense core vesicles contain catecholamines or serotonin at a synapse.

33. a. e.

Golgi tendon organs take part in the inverse stretch reflex whereas the stretch reflex requires muscle spindles. Gamma stimulation shortens the intrafusal fibres, thereby deforming the annulospiral endings. This initiates impulses in the Ia afferents which may lead to reflex contraction of the extrafusal fibres. The pathway is therefore indirect. Central delay is a minimum of 0.5 s. In the knee jerk the delay is 0.6–0.9 s. The law of Bell–Magendie states that in the spinal cord the dorsal roots are sensory and the ventral roots are motor.

34. b. d.
The area sensitive to acetylcholine increases – one cause of denervation supersensitivity. The number of receptors may increase or more of the existing ones are activated. The nerve undergoes Wallerian degeneration. Strong electrical stimulation producing contraction against a load will delay atrophy. Denervated muscles usually show contracture.

35. a. c. d. e.
Under normal conditions, absorption of cerebrospinal fluid is proportional to the pressure. At an average cerebrospinal fluid pressure, production and absorption are essentially equal. As pressure increases, absorption increases linearly. However below a pressure of approximately 70 mm, cerebrospinal fluid absorption stops. It flows from the fourth ventricle into the cisterna magna via the single midline foramen of Magendie and the two lateral foramina of Lusckha. The post lumbar headache is due to the unsupported brain stretching the neurovascular bundles. This can be relieved by restoring fluid support with isotonic solution. In communicating external hydrocephalus the reabsorptive capacity of the arachnoid villi is decreased, hence there is an accumulation of fluid within the ventricular system. This is in contrast to internal or non-communicating hydrocephalus, which occurs due to an obstruction in the outflow of cerebrospinal fluid or within the ventricular system. Hence fluid accumulates proximal to the block.

36. a. e.
Critical damping ensures that tympanic vibration stops almost immediately after the sound wave stops. The reaction time of the tympanic reflex is 40–160 ms and is too slow to protect the ear adequately. The normal range of audible sound is 20 Hz–20 kHz. Convection currents causing movements of the cupula evoke the

response to caloric stimuli. Bone conduction in a normal subject is masked by environmental noise. In a patient with conduction deafness (who cannot hear environmental noise), bone conduction appears better than in a normal subject. This is the basis of the Schwabach test.

37. c. e.
Gamma-aminobutyric acid and glycine are inhibitory neurotransmitters.

Dopamine and other monoamines (e.g. 5-hydroxytryptamine) are also inhibitory neurotransmitters.

38. a. b. c. d.
Cardiac output is governed by the product of heart rate and stroke volume. Stroke volume is increased by increasing the preload, reducing afterload and increasing the contractility of heart muscle. The normal cardiac output is approximately 5 l/min which is effectively the same as the venous return to the right atrium, as explained by Starling's law of the heart. An arteriovenous fistula increases venous return and so increases preload. In the trained athlete, the heart may increase in size by 50% so cardiac output may increase to 20 l/min. This may increase to 35 l/min with increase autonomic stimulation. The normal systemic filling pressure is 7 mmHg. This may be doubled by an increase in the blood volume of 15–30%. Measurement of cardiac output by the Fick principle requires a knowledge of the arteriovenous oxygen difference and total oxygen consumption.

39. All
In a normal electrocardiogram the PR interval represents atrial depolarization and conduction through the atrioventricular node. It is usually 0.12–0.20 s in duration and is therefore increased during atrioventricular nodal block. The QRS complex represents ventricular depolarization and atrial repolarization and is usually 0.08–0.12 s and may be increased in any form of bundle branch block. The ST interval represents ventricular repolarization and hence the refractory period of the ventricular myocardium.

40. b. c.
At the onset of moderate exercise there is an abrupt increase in

ventilation rate. Shift of the oxygen dissociation curve and greater blood flow in exercise allow a 100-fold increase in metabolic rate. The RQ rises due to the increased production of carbon dioxide. The pH stays the same in mild and moderate exercise but falls in strenuous exercise. Cardiac output rises at the most seven-fold.

41. a. d. e.
Isometric ventricular relaxation occurs when the aortic valve closes and the ventricle is then a closed cavity.

The ventricle ejects about 60 ml of blood during each contraction. It does not empty completely. Thus the difference between the end-diastolic volume and the end-systolic volume is the stroke volume.

42. a. c. e.
The main baroreceptor site in humans is in the carotid sinus. The low-pressure receptors are stimulated by an increase in the blood volume in the right atrium and great veins.

43. a. c. e.
The compliance is increased in emphysema and decreased in pulmonary congestion.

44. All
Gravity has the effect of reducing the central blood pool by as much as 400 ml. The stroke volume is also reduced by as much as 40%. Since the stroke volume determines the cardiac output:

Cardiac output = stroke volume × heart rate

the cardiac output is also reduced.

There is a reflex component of the response to postural change. The heart rate is increased in order to minimize the fall in the cardiac output. Also the total peripheral resistance is increased by as much as 25% in order to maintain the blood pressure. This reflex is diminished by prolonged recumbency.

45. b. c. d. e.
Osteoporosis is the loss of bone density due to excessive absorption of calcium and phosphorus from the bone. It affects predominantly postmenopausal women and affects cortical and trabecular bone equally. There is usually no derangement of the bone biochemistry,

which is in marked contrast to the results obtained in Paget's disease, osteomalacia and primary hyperparathyroidism. Both hypothyroidism and hyperthyroidism directly stimulate the bone turnover which may cause osteoporosis. Biphosphonates, of which etidronate is an example, are used to help prevent bone resorption as they act to inhibit the osteoclasts.

46. b. d. e.
Analgesics can be simply classed as narcotic or non-narcotic. Aspirin and paracetamol are both examples of non-narcotic analgesics. Aspirin and similar drugs inhibit the cycloxygenase enzyme, thereby diminishing the production of endoperoxides and prostaglandins from arachidonate. These prostaglandins lower the firing threshold of primary afferent polymodal C fibres, hence sensitizing nerve endings to the effects of bradykinin and histamine released in response to injury. Paracetamol is a more potent inhibitor of brain cycloxygenase and has little anti-inflammatory action. The narcotic analgesics such as morphine, diamorphine, codeine and pethidine are thought to act on opiate receptors which have been studied in detail. There are five different subtypes: the μ-receptor seems to be concerned with central pain mechanisms and is the receptor for the natural alkaloid morphine. They are found both within the brain and also in the spinal cord. Codeine is a semisynthetic drug, as is diamorphine. Pethidine is a fully synthetic narcotic.

47. b. c. d.
Positively inotropic refers to the situation where a chemical or drug has a positive effect on the contractility of the cardiac muscle. Dopamine exerts its affect via the β-receptors, so causing an increase in cyclic adenosine monophosphate. A similar situation is also caused by theophylline and glucagon as these inhibit the breakdown of cyclic adenosine monophosphate. Nifedipine is a calcium channel blocker and is therefore negatively inotropic. Adenosine, an endogenous nucleoside, is negatively inotropic and has increasingly been used as an alternative to direct-current cardioversion in terminating paroxysmal supraventricular tachycardias.

48. b.

It is the Sertoli cells which are responsible for supporting and nourishing the spermatozoa. They also secrete inhibin, which exerts a negative feedback effect on follicle-stimulating hormone secretion.

The Leydig cells are responsible for testosterone production. Testosterone produces a negative feedback effect on luteinizing hormone secretion.

For spermatogenesis to be initiated, the Sertoli cells must be primed with follicle-stimulating hormone, not testosterone. However testosterone is required for the maintenance of spermatogenesis.

49. a. b. c. e.

Progesterone exhibits a negative feedback action on luteinizing hormone secretion and is responsible for the decrease in its concentration in the secretory phase of the cycle. Only oestradiol at high concentration can exhibit a positive feedback action on follicle-stimulating hormone and luteinizing hormone secretion.

50. b. d. e.

Usually 65% of sodium ions are reabsorbed actively in the proximal tubule followed by chloride and then water. Very little sodium is absorbed in the thin segments of the loop of Henle; however in the diluting segment of the early distal tubule, chloride is actively reabsorbed, followed by sodium. Potassium is predominantly reabsorbed in a similar way to sodium; however, in the distal tubules under the influence of aldosterone, it may be secreted actively into the late distal tubules and collecting ducts. Hydrogen ions are secreted more generally into the filtrate along the tubules. The countercurrent multiplier system of the loop of Henle is important for concentrating urine. This involves creating a high osmolality in the medullary interstitial fluid such that the water may be reabsorbed from a collecting duct at it passes through it. One of the mechanisms increasing this osmolality is the reabsorption of at least 50% of the urea as it passes down a collecting duct. The countercurrent exchange system of the vasa recta prevents removal of the ions, providing this increased osmolality.

51. a. b. c. e.
Vasa recta are high-resistance vessels.

The kidney contains the hydroxylase enzyme which converts 25-hydroxyvitamin D to 1,25 dihydroxyvitamin D. In chronic renal failure, oestomalcia may occur due to failure of conversion to the more active form of vitamin D.

52. All
If there are inadequate calories in the diet, ingested fats and proteins are used to provide energy. Insulin is anabolic when glucose is available. Androgens and oestrogens are both anabolic for protein and increase the response of growth hormone to stimuli such as insulin. Thyroid hormones have a permissive action on growth hormone and its secretion.

53. a. c. d.
It is important during the process of starvation that the metabolism of protein is prevented for as long as possible. This is achieved by maintaining the glucose levels as well as switching to the metabolism of fats. Gluconeogenesis is stimulated by glucagon and adrenaline, while glycogenolysis is stimulated mainly by glucagon. As time goes on, deamination in the kidney becomes important in providing substrates for the gluconeogenesis process which may even start to occur in the kidney itself. Lipolysis is stimulated by growth hormone, so providing free fatty acids which may either be metabolized directly by β-oxidation or converted to ketones in the liver for later use, by all the organs except the renal medulla and erythrocytes. The brain itself may use a portion of ketones late in starvation. Conversion of thyroxine to the largely inactive reversed tri-iodothyronine also occurs as the glucose levels drop.

54. a. d.
There is increased breakdown of fat to free acids and glycerol and a decrease in basal metabolic rate (BMR) and body temperature. Oxygen consumption falls to begin with, but rises later. Membrane potentials tend to fall, perhaps due to lack of adenosine triphosphate and other energy stores. Gluconeogenesis and low insulin levels decrease the glucose tolerance.

55. b. e.
Tri-iodothyronine binds to nuclear receptors. In hyperthyroidism the rate of cholesterol removal is greater than the rate of synthesis. Cholesterol levels therefore decrease. Albumin has the greatest *capacity* for thyroxine binding, but thyroid-binding globulin has the greatest *affinity*. Some 67% of thyroxine is bound to thyroid-binding globulin. Thyroid hormones raise the level of 2,3-DPG in erythrocytes, thereby shifting the dissociation curve to the right.

56. a. b. d.
Gastrin increases gastric motility, with a mild effect on the small bowel. 5-Hydroxytryptamine, in association with the carcinoid syndrome, causes diarrhoea. Secretin has a mild inhibitory effect on most of the gastrointestinal tract. In general terms, the sympathetic nervous system has an inhibitory effect on the intestinal tract whereas the parasympathetic nervous system has a stimulatory effect.

57. b. c.
Urea is predominantly formed in the liver, therefore there is a marked drop in this substance after total hepatectomy. The urea is thought to help remove ammonia which therefore rises and is thought to be a major component of hepatic coma. Liver is a major store of glycogen and producer of albumin, therefore hypoglycaemia and hypoalbuminaemia are common. The majority of gamma-globulins are formed by plasma cells therefore there is no marked drop in their level.

58. a. b. e.
The main function of the colon is absorption of water, sodium and minerals. Sodium is actively absorbed out of the colon, closely followed by water down the osmotic gradient created. Potassium and bicarbonate are secreted. Material is moved along the colon in three main ways: segmentation helps to mix the contents; peristalsis helps propel them towards the rectum; mass action contraction moves the material from one portion of the colon to another. Mass action contraction only occurs in the colon, where there is simultaneous contraction of smooth muscle over large confluent areas. These movements in the colon are coordinated by a colonic slow wave, whose frequency increases along the colon from 2/min

at the ileocaecal valve to 6/min in the sigmoid colon. Mucus is secreted in the colon but there are almost no enzymes.

59. c.
Hydrochloric acid and intrinsic factor are secreted by the parietal cells. The chief cells are responsible for secretion of pepsinogens.
   Gastrin is secreted by G cells in the antrum.

60. All
Pancreatic secretion consists of inorganic and organic fractions. The inorganic fraction is stimulated by secretin and its effect is potentiated by gastrin and cholecystokinin. The organic fraction is stimulated by cholecystokinin, which also causes the gall bladder to contract.

61. a. b.
In multifactorial inheritance, several genes may have an additive effect or there may be an interaction between genetic and environmental factors. The incidence of such conditions among relatives is higher than in the general population. Familial polyposis coli is an autosomal dominant condition, congenital adrenal hyperplasia is autosomal recessive and haemophilia is due to X-linked recessive inheritance.

62. a. d. e.
Class 2 molecules of the human leukocyte antigen system play an important role in antigen recognition by T cells.

63. a. b. c.
Haemochromatosis affects men more than women: presumably women are protected by menstruation against the accumulation of iron.
   'Sago' spleen refers to the appearance of the spleen resulting from the deposition of amyloid.

64. a. c. d.
Pannus formation is a feature of rheumatoid arthritis. The subchondral cysts are actually pseudocysts filled with myxomatous fibrous tissue. Synovial proliferation occurs as a feature of rheumatoid arthritis.

65. a. c. d.
Adult respiratory distress syndrome is characterized by non-cardiac pulmonary infiltrates, respiratory distress and refractory hypoxaemia. Common causes are shock, septicaemia, burns and fat embolism. Supra-added infection with resistant organisms such as *Pseudomonas aeruginosa* is a common cause of death in this disease. Treatment is difficult and usually involves supportive care with ventilation and treatment of any known cause. Steroids have been used but are of disputed benefit.

66. b. c. e.
Subacute bacterial endocarditis usually affects diseased hearts such as are found in congenital anomalies or rheumatic fever. It is usually caused by low-virulence organisms such as *Streptococcus viridans* but may also be caused by the enterococci – *Haemophilus* and *Coxiella* species. The mitral valve is usually affected most, or in combination with the aortic valve; other valves are rarely affected in isolation. The damage caused tends to be slow in progressing but may cause severe functional disturbances. The acute form of endocarditis tends to be caused by virulent organisms such as *Staphylococcus aureus* or pneumococcus and tends to affect structurally normal hearts or ones which have recently undergone cardiac surgery. Drug addicts and alcoholics are particularly at risk and there may be extra cardiac foci of infection.

67. a. b. d.
In 70% of cases there is thymic hyperplasia and in 10% there is a thymic neoplasm. The antibodies involved are of the immunoglobulin G type. Infections, aminoglycosides and magnesium salt enemas may provoke a myasthenic crisis. Statement e describes Eaton–Lambert syndrome in which weakness improves after repeated muscle contraction.

68. d. e.
Candidiasis is caused by a yeast. Broad-spectrum antibiotics which upset the usual balance of flora often result in proliferation of *Candida*. In the healthy subject, small numbers of *Candida* are found in the mouth and bowel. Candidiasis is commoner in diabetics and is a cause of intertrigo. Treatment is with clotrimazole or ketoconazole.

69. a. c. d. e.
Gas gangrene is caused by Gram-positive anaerobic spore-forming bacteria which are found in faeces (the spores are found in soil). Any area contaminated with faeces will harbour the organism. Therefore the perineum and, occasionally, the vagina may house the organism. Gangrene, by definition, is necrosis with putrefaction. High-dose penicillin and hyperbaric oxygen together with antiserum and adequate debridement are indicated.

70. b. d.
Herpes simplex viruses types 1 and 2 produce recurrent herpetic vesicles in the oral and genital regions.

Varicella-zoster virus produces chickenpox on first exposure. It lies dormant in the dorsal root ganglion and commonly in the trigeminal sensory ganglion. Reactivation produces shingles.

71. b. d.
Hepatitis A virus is a small RNA virus.

Hepatic cirrhosis results from infection with hepatitis B, non-A, non-B and C viruses, not from hepatitis A virus.

72. a. b. d. e.
Actinomyces israelii spreads along fascial planes and occasionally via blood but not via lymphatics.

73. All

74. d. e.
Exotoxins are predominantly protein and may be used to form toxoids. They are heat-labile, of high potency and have an unspecific effect on a variety of tissues: all tend to be different. In contrast, endotoxins are lipid in form, heat-stable and are of much lower potency.

75. b. c. d. e.
In metabolic acidosis hydrogen ions are lost in the kidney and therefore potassium ions are retained. There is also an increased loss of potassium from the cells. Carbonic anhydrase inhibitors such as acetozolamide inhibit sodium reabsorption in the proximal tubules, therefore there is an increased load in the distal tubules where it is reabsorbed at the expense of potassium. Pyloric stenosis

leads to a loss of potassium via two mechanisms. The first is directly in the vomitus with the resulting alkalosis leading the hydrogen ion-sparing in the kidney at the expense of potassium loss. Alkalosis also drives potassium into the cells. The large amount of mucus lost in the villous papilloma is rich in potassium.

76. b. c.
Hypokalaemic alkalosis occurs in pyloric stenosis. There is paradoxical acid urine excretion due to excretion of hydrogen and potassium ions in order to conserve the depleted sodium pool.

The alkalosis causes a shift of the ionized calcium ions to the unionized state which results in tetany. The total calcium concentration is not affected.

Urea concentration rises due to dehydration and renal impairment.

77. a. e.
Albumin is a protein which has a half-life which is over 20 days. Its concentration in the plasma compartment must be greter than that in the interstitial compartment under normal conditions, so preventing oedema according to Starling's law. Increased acute-phase proteins in acute inflammation may lead to hypoalbuminaemia.

78. a. d. e.
The human immunodeficiency virus infects the T-helper cells.

It is the T lymphocytes which form rosettes with sheep red blood cells. B lymphocytes have Fc receptors, C3b receptors and immunoglobulins on their surface.

79. b. c. d. e.
In macrocytosis there is usually a mean cell volume of over 96 fl. Two of the commonest causes of macrocytosis are vitamin B_{12} deficiency, e.g. in pernicious anaemia, and folate deficiency which may occur in treatment with anticonvulsants, haematological diseases with increased red cell production, e.g. haemolytic anaemias and poor intake due either to anorexia or poor diet. Other important causes of macrocytosis include excessive alcohol ingestion, liver disease, hypothyroidism, reticulocytosis and aplastic anaemia.

80. b. c.
Platelets are derived by cytoplasmic pinching from megakaryocytes
and hence have no nucleus. They are 0.2–0.4 µ in size and have a
mean life span of 7–10 days. Some 60–75% are contained in the
circulation and 25% in the spleen. They contain two types of
granules: dense granules, which contain non-proteins such as ADP
serotonin and 5-hydroxytryptamine and alpha granules which
contain proteins such as clotting factors and platelet-derived
growth factor. There is an extensive canalicular system on the
surface, important for increasing the surface area for release and
chemical signals. In von Willebrand's disease there is a defect of
platelet adhesion due to the failure of synthesis of factor VIII:R.

81. a. b.
In pericanalicular fibroadenomas, epithelial arrangement is pre-
served, whereas in the intracanalicular variety seen in a slightly old
age group, there are blunt fingers of fibrous tissue distorting
epithelium into branching clefts. A cystosarcoma phylloides tumour
is an example of a giant intracanalicular fibroadenoma. Family
history is an important aetiological factor in ductal carcinoma
which is three times as common as intralobular carcinoma. There is
approximately a 1:5 chance of lobular carcinoma being bilateral
and the degree of lymphocytic response to tumour has an important
bearing on the prognosis of the tumour – the greater the response,
the better the prognosis.

82. All
The epithelium of bronchus, gall bladder and bladder may all
undergo squamous metaplasia as a result of stones, irritation or
chronic infection. The prostate does similarly, under the excessive
oestrogens used to treat carcinoma. The acid-secreting gastric lining
may be changed to a mucus-secreting lining of intestinal type in
association with atrophic gastritis and gastric atrophy.

83. a. c.
M proteins are found in multiple myeloma, malignant lymphoma,
Waldenström's macroglobulinaemia and heavy chain disease. There
is a proliferation of plasma cells which produce immunoglobulin G
(55% of cases), A (23%) or M in the case of Waldenström's. Bence
Jones proteins precipitate on heating to 60–80°C and redissolve at

higher temperatures. Hypercalcaemia rather than hypocalcaemia is a common feature.

84. a. b. c. e.
Adenocarcinoma is commonest in the lower third and may spread from gastric epithelium, but more commonly spreads from a Barrett mucosa. Carcinoma may be preceded by varying degrees of dysplasia. Tylosis is an inherited condition in which there is keratosis of the palms and soles with a predisposition to the development of oesophageal carcinoma. The commonest benign tumour is the leiomyoma.

85. a. c. d. e.
Adenocarcinoma of the prostate gland typically causes osteoblastic lesions. It is testosterone-dependent and therefore is treated by antitestosterone drugs such as cyproterone acetate.

86. b. c. d. e.
Wound healing is affected by many factors. Increasing the temperature surrounding a wound by 10°C is said to double the rate of healing. Ionizing radiation affects vascularity and inhibits wound contracture. Protein deficiency and hypovitaminosis are well-recognized causes of poor healing. Zinc therapy is only thought to help when serum levels are low.

87. a. b. e.
C-reactive protein (an acute-phase protein) is so named because it reacts as a precipitin with the C polysaccharide of pneumococcus. Its level is raised in pneumococcal pneumonia, neoplasia, systemic lupus erythematosus, leukaemias, inflammatory bowel disease and viral infections. A rise in the erythroycte sedimentation rate is usually accompanied by a rise in C-reactive protein levels.

88. d. e.
Myofibroblasts are important in wound contraction but collagen contraction is not. Vitamin C is essential for normal collagen formation and therefore deficiency impedes normal healing. A skin graft containing dermis will prevent contraction.

89. a. b.
Papillary necrosis results from chronic ingestion of aspirin/

phenacetin, diabetes mellitus and sickle cell anaemia.

90. All

Approaching the *viva voce* examination

Candidates worry, sometimes needlessly, about the vivas predominantly due to fear of the unknown. This section is designed to provide examples of viva questions that have been asked in the last 4 years as well as some insight into the format of the vivas.

You already know that the different sections of the examination are marked on the basis that 12 counts as a pass, less than 12 is a fail and more than 12 is very good. At the beginning of the viva you will have a score of 12 and thereon can gain or lose marks according to your performance. If you can do well in the viva and score 13 it will make up for that 11 you scraped in the MCQ. Likewise, a 13 in the MCQ can see you through in the face of a poor show in the viva. You know that you should aim for a total of 36 in each discipline (anatomy, physiology and pathology) in order to pass the whole examination.

In the event of a candidate scoring 35, the marks are scrutinized and any examiner who gave you an 11 is asked to justify that mark and it is at this stage that the candidate can be brought up to the pass level. Thus, for borderline cases, the examiners do their best to award a pass if the marks allow it. This runs against the beliefs of most candidates.

The examiners are usually fair, with the few exceptions expected at any examination. If you are struggling, most will help you to extract the information required. If you find yourself answering a series of questions incorrectly try keeping quiet and letting them prompt you with some clues. Endless wrong answers can only mean failure!

It is important to be confident, whether answering the question or saying you do not know. Be careful if you are the sort of person who guesses the answers. Even a confident guesser can get it wrong and examiners will spot you very easily.

Smart dress is essential. It conveys the impression that you are fit to deal with members of the public as a representative of the College of Surgeons and it shows that you are taking the examination seriously.

It is important when reading the questions in this section to use them as examples only. It is impossible to convey in printed form the flow of each viva. What appears to be a very difficult question may have been asked only if the candidate was doing very well and often serves as a starter for more searching ones. The manner in which you begin your answer is very important. Try to think quietly for a moment before you begin. During this time think how you will structure the answer. A sensible structure shows the examiner that you are able to think clearly and logically. If you have no idea what the question is getting at then you can either say that you don't know the answer or you can talk in general terms about the key words in the question. The examiner will soon redirect you if you are on the wrong track. Be prepared to draw a diagram or graph if you are asked to. In our experience volunteering to draw a diagram when not asked to had dire consequences.

Finally, do not worry. It is amazing what answers you will be able to put together in the heat of the moment. Good luck!

Anatomy vivas

Histology slides

Gastrointestinal tract
Tongue, oesophagus, gastro-oesophageal junction, duodenum, ileum, colon, anorectal junction.

Reproductive tissue
Uterus, uterine cervix, testis, vas deferens, ovary, fallopian tubes.

Muscle
Cardiac muscle, smooth muscle (intestine), skeletal muscle, tongue muscle.

Other tissues
Salivary glands, pancreas, liver, kidney, ureter, bladder, developing bone, skin of lip, cartilage, tonsil, lymph node, thymus, thyroid.

Viva questions

1. What are the histological differences between vas deferens and ureter?
   What structures pass through the following skull foramina: stylomastoid, jugular, spinosum?
   What structures form the anterior and posterior pillars of the oropharynx?
   What is the structure of the eustachian tube? What mechanisms open its pharyngeal orifice?
   Name and point out the dural sinuses. What is the direction of blood flow in them?
   What structures lie in the cavernous sinus?
   What is the course of the facial nerve?

2. What are the contents of the adductor canal?
   Show me how you would find the obturator nerve in the thigh (on a prosection).
   Identify the superior mesenteric artery. What is its embryology and how does it come to lie anterior to the uncinate lobe of the pancreas?
   How does a long bone develop?

3. Candidate shown a skull X-ray: What is the age of the patient? At what age do the permanent teeth appear? Point out and name the sutures.
   What are the branches of the superficial femoral artery?
   At what level does the common carotid artery bifurcate? How would you distinguish the internal from the external carotid artery?
   Describe the first rib and its muscle attachments What nerves are related to it?

4. What are the ligaments of the hip joint? What are the dangers of hip dislocation?
   What is the blood supply of the femoral head?
   Describe typical features of a thoracic vertebra.
   Candidate shown the os innominatum: Describe its muscle attachments.
   Candidate given the femur, tibia and patella: Show the attachment of the joint capsule of the knee. Is the patella from the same side of the body as the femur?
   How much weight is transmitted from the patellar tendon?
   How is arthroscopy performed?

5. Candidate given an articulated hand: Name the carpal bones.
   What are the contents of the carpal tunnel?
   Candidate shown prosected foot: What are the contents of the sinus tarsi? What muscles attach to the fifth metatarsal bone?
   What is the action of peroneus longus?
   What happens at the level of T4–5?
   What comprises the floor of the mouth?
   Identify the salivary glands (on a prosection).
   What are the strap muscles? What is their function and innervation?

6. Candidate given a clavicle: Tell me all you know about that bone.
   Candidate shown computed tomography scan at level of T12/L1: Identify as many structures as you can.

7. Candidate taken to live model: Show me the transpyloric plane. What structures lie in it?
   Demonstrate the anatomical snuff box.
   How would you show the brachioradialis muscle in this model?
   Examine the knee joint and show the joint line.

8. Tell me about the mandible and how it changes from newborn to pensioner.
   How does the testis end up in the scrotum?
   What does gubernaculum mean?

Physiology vivas

1. What is the physiology of nervousness? Describe:
   The effect of adrenaline on the feeling of hunger.
   The effects of steroids on blood sugar and the immune system.
   The other hormones involved in stress.
   The effects of pure alpha and pure beta receptor stimulation.

2. In discussing splenectomy:
   What are the effects on the blood film?
   What are the reasons for pneumococcal sensitivity?
   Describe the drugs which influence platelet survival
   What is the mechanism of platelet function?
   What are the contents of platelets?
   Describe the hormones acting on blood calcium levels.
   What is the role of calcitonin?

3. What is shock?
   Describe the physiological response to removing 1 litre of blood slowly (over a period of 10 min).
   Describe Starling's forces and the causes of oedema.

4. What is the function of the gall bladder?
   Describe its hormonal control.
   What is gastrin? Describe its function.
   How does one measure glomerular filtration rate, renal plasma flow and clearance?
   Describe the relation of insulin and glucose levels to the dumping syndrome.
   Draw a graph to represent this.

5. Tell me about splanchnic circulation.
   What is the arrangement of vessels in the bowel wall?
   Draw the structure of an intestinal villus.
   How does the arrangement of vessels help the function of the villus?
   Describe which solutes are transported to set up the osmotic gradient.
   What is the pressure in the hepatic portal vein, the hepatic artery, the hepatic veins and the sinusoids?
   What is the significance of these pressure differences?
   What is the detailed histological arrangement in the sinusoids?

6. Classify the causes of jaundice.

At what level of bilirubin does jaundice become clinically evident?

Describe the investigation of the patient and the interpretation of the results.

What is Courvoisier's law?

What are the complications of jaundice?

What is hepatorenal syndrome? What preoperative measures help prevent it?

What precipitates hepatic encephalopathy? How is it treated?

What single biochemical test is the best indicator of liver function?

7. Describe the cardiac muscle cell.

   How does it differ from skeletal muscle?

   Draw the action potential and contraction curve.

   Describe in detail the specific permeability changes and their consequences.

   Describe:

   The role of calcium in muscle contraction

   The molecular mechanism of tetany in hypocalcaemia.

   Does a decrease in calcium stop the heart in systole or diastole?

   How does the T tubular system differ in cardiac and skeletal muscle?

   Describe the molecular mechanism of skeletal muscle contraction. Include a diagram of the filaments.

8. Tell me everything you know about acute pancreatitis.

   Discuss the complications of acute pancreatitis.

9. Describe the molecular events involved in the synthesis of thyroxine.

   Discuss the control of the thyroid hormones.

   How are the hormones transported? What proportion is bound?

   Which drugs control thyroid hormone levels and how?

   Describe the effects of thyroxine.

10. What is the cardiovascular response before, during and after clamping of the aorta?

    If a patient has a groin stab wound, how quickly does he or she die?

11. Tell me about temperature regulation in general terms.
    How am I losing heat now?
    What is radiation?
    What is the rate of temperature rise in the absence of regulation?
    Describe the metabolism of iron.
    How is it absorbed and what is its function in the body?
    Where is iron stored?

12. What is the cardiovascular response to fracture of the femoral shaft in a 30-year-old?

13. Tell me the injuries caused by a stab wound to the left side of the chest.
    What is pneumothorax?
    Why does air enter the chest?
    What are the advantages and disadvantages of the changes in intrathoracic pressure which occur in normal breathing?
    What is a hormone?

14. Let's talk about oxygen delivery.
    Draw the oxygen dissociation curve. How does its shape help deliver oxygen to the tissues?
    What is the partial pressure of oxygen in: a mitochondrion; an exercising cell.
    Draw the oxygen dissociation curve in exercising muscle.
    In what other ways can oxygen delivery be increased?
    Describe the tendon jerk.
    Describe the function of the muscle spindle.

15. Give some examples of hypertension which is amenable to surgery.
    Describe the mechanisms involved in each example.
    What happens in renal artery stenosis? Why doesn't the affected kidney autoregulate?
    What drugs can be used to treat hypertension?
    How does methyldopa act?
    Give an example of a ganglion blocker.
    How do calcium antagonists work?
    What is surfactant and how does it help in the alveoli?
    How would you manage a patient with no surfactant? What oxygen concentration would you use in ventilation?

16. Discuss the effects of excision of the duodenum.
    Discuss total parenteral nutrition.
    What can be learnt from a lumbar puncture?
    What is the composition of cerebrospinal fluid and its pressure?
    What parts of the brain lie outside the blood–brain barrier?
    What are the functions of these parts?
    Describe the circulation in the anterior pituitary.
    Define an endocrine cell as opposed to a neuron.
    Name some neurotransmitters. Which are excitatory?

Pathology vivas

1. What are the functions of formalin in tissue fixation?
   What are the changes after cell death? What are the nuclear changes?
   What are the causes of macrocytosis? What are the functions of folate and vitamin B_{12}?
   What are the causes of deficiency of folate and vitamin B_{12}?
   What are the causes and effects of hypernatraemia?
   What are oncogenes? What is their relevance in oncogenesis? Give examples of oncogenes.
   What chromosomal changes are seen in neoplastic tissue?
   Classify chemical carcinogens. What is their mechanism of action?

2. What is a transfusion reaction?
   List the complications of blood transfusion.
   What is a polyp?
   Describe different types of polyp.
   Describe using diagrams Dukes' classification. What is its practical relevence?

3. What is pus?
   How does one culture organisms from pus and blood?
   What organisms cause wound infection?
   Define bacteraemia, pyaemia and septicaemia.
   What is subacute bacterial endocarditis (SBE)?
   What is a fistula? What are the causes of a fistula and what mechanisms maintain it?
   What is a diverticulum? What is diverticular disease?

4. How are bacteria classified?
   What are the differences between Gram-positive and Gram-negative organisms?
   How is a Gram stain performed?
   What is the composition of endotoxin?
   Which is the antigenic component of endotoxin?
   What are staphylococci? Is *Staphylococcus epidermidis* important as a pathogen?
   What determines virulence?
   What are scalded skin syndrome and toxic shock syndrome?
   What is the treatment of these syndromes and what are their histological features?
   What are the causes of endotoxic shock?

Can endotoxin be measured in the circulation? Name the quantitative test.

What are the causes and effects of hepatitis?

What are immunological markers of hepatitis? What indicates high infectivity in hepatitis B?

What are the complications of hepatitis?

What are the high-risk groups and how would you deal with them in an operation?

5. Classify the causes of lymphadenopathy and give examples of them.

   What are the changes that are seen in a lymph node during malignancy?

   What cellular functions and interactions occur in a lymph node?

   What are the causes of cervical lymphadenopathy?

   What is the commonest cause of localized cervical lymphadenopathy?

   How are lymphomas classified?

   Tell me about testicular tumours.

6. Tell me how tumours are classified and staged.

   What are the effects of tumours on the host.

   Name some tumour markers. Of what use is carcinoembryonic antigen?

   What was the first tumour marker to be discovered?

   How do tumours spread?

   What are the commonest sites of metastases and what are the usual primary sites?

   What tumours spread to bone? Which cause lytic and which cause sclerotic changes?

   What are the effects of bone metastases at cellular level?

   What is a pathological fracture and how would you treat one?

7. Tell me about antibodies.

   Classify hypersensitivity reactions and give examples of each.

   What is gas gangrene? What causes it?

   What is Paget's disease of the breast? What histological changes are seen? What clinical signs help to differentiate it from eczema?

   What is amyloid? What effects does it have?

8. What are the differences between benign and malignant

tumours?
Tell me all you know about skin tumours.

9. What is osteomyelitis? What are its causes?
What sort of people get salmonella osteomyelitis?
What are the effects of osteomyelitis?
What gross changes are seen in the affected bone?

10. Tell me about suture materials.
How do they decay?
What difference is there between natural and synthetic materials?
What is carcinoma-*in-situ*?

11. Compare and contrast osteomalacia and osteoporosis.
What are the causes and effects of immunosuppression?
What sorts of diverticula do you know? What are their causes and effects?

12. Define neoplasm, hyperplasia, hypertrophy, dysplasia and heteroplasia.
What are the causes and effects of venous thrombosis?
What are the different types of leukaemia?

13. Tell me about renal failure.
What is the pathology of prerenal failure?
What are the causes of postrenal failure?
How can cancer of the prostate cause postrenal failure without obstructing bladder outflow?
Tell me about immunocytochemistry. How is it useful?

14. Define dialysis. What types do you know?
What are the complications of peritoneal dialysis?
What organisms may infect the apparatus? What precautions are taken to prevent infection?
What organisms cause infections of the ear?
What causes malignant otitis externa?
What do bacterial capsules do?

15. Tell me about macrophages.
What is a granuloma? How would you classify granulomas?
In what diseases are granulomas found?

16. Draw me a diagram of a healing wound. Which layer is proliferating?
    How do the cells migrate?
    Where do the macrophages come from?
    What is collagen? How is it synthesized? What is its structure?
    Do you know any defects of collagen synthesis?
    Tell me about the clinical presentation of vitamin C deficiency.
    Tell me about the effects of steroids on wound healing.
    What is the difference between acute and chronic inflammation?

17. Give some examples of hyperplasia.
    What are the effects of parathyroid hyperplasia?
    What is the effect of this process on bone?
    Define embolism. What types of embolus do you know?
    What are the pathological effects of pulmonary embolism?

18. Tell me about calculi.
    How and why do calculi form?
    What are renal stones made of?
    Are oxalate stones common? What shape are they?
    What types of sterilization do you know?
    Give examples of chemicals used in sterilization.
    At what temperature and pressure does an autoclave work?
    How do you tell that an autoclave is functioning effectively?

19. What is an aneurysm? What causes an aneurysm? Give some examples.
    What are the causes and effects of hypocalcaemia?
    What organisms may be grown from a throat swab?
    What is the typical blood picture of bacterial pharyngitis?
    What is the blood picture in glandular fever?
    What are the causes of agranulocytosis?
    What is the blood picture in acute leukaemia?